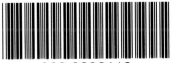

Listening
to Pain

A Clinician's Guide

to Improving Pain

Management Through

Better Communication

Scott M. Fishman, MD
Professor and Chief
Division of Pain Medicine
University of California, Davis

OXFORD
UNIVERSITY PRESS

OXFORD
UNIVERSITY PRESS

Oxford University Press, Inc., publishes works that further
Oxford University's objective of excellence
in research, scholarship, and education.

Oxford New York
Auckland   Cape Town   Dar es Salaam   Hong Kong   Karachi
Kuala Lumpur   Madrid   Melbourne   Mexico City   Nairobi
New Delhi   Shanghai   Taipei   Toronto

With offices in
Argentina   Austria   Brazil   Chile   Czech Republic   France   Greece
Guatemala   Hungary   Italy   Japan   Poland   Portugal   Singapore
South Korea   Switzerland   Thailand   Turkey   Ukraine   Vietnam

Copyright © 2012 Scott M. Fishman

Published by Oxford University Press, Inc.
198 Madison Avenue, New York, New York 10016
www.oup.com

Oxford is a registered trademark of Oxford University Press

Library of Congress Cataloging-in-Publication Data

Fishman, Scott
Listening to pain : a clinician's guide to improving pain management through
better communication / Scott M. Fishman.
    p. ; cm.
  ISBN 978-0-19-989198-6 (pbk. : alk. paper)
I. Title.
[DNLM: 1. Pain—therapy. 2. Clinician-Patient Relations. WL 704]
616'.0472—dc23

Printed in the United States of America on acid-free paper

This book is dedicated to the memory of Jan Aaron.

Contents

Listening
to Pain

Introduction
The Healing Art of Communication

When clinicians first learn that my specialty is pain medicine, they tend to respond with sympathy, bordering on pity. "What a way to practice medicine," they say, shaking their head in condolence, or else, "Pain patients are … such a *pain*! How do you do it day after day?"

I tell them honestly that pain medicine is the most challenging *and rewarding* field I could imagine. Chronic pain is the consummate mind-body disorder, so treating pain makes complex demands on the mind, the imagination, and the heart of the practitioner. On any given day in the pain clinic, I am called upon to be a medical detective, a psychiatrist, and a chaplain.

The biggest challenge and the greatest reward of pain medicine is that it requires me to connect with my patients on the most personal level—where they suffer and hurt. Like most doctors I know, my decision to enter the medical profession began with an altruistic desire to relieve suffering. So much of the way medicine is practiced today conspires to distance us from our idealistic beginnings as clinicians. We're all working within the constraints of a healthcare system that's long on bureaucratic red tape and increasingly short on the most precious resource of all: time. Treating patients in pain doesn't liberate you from those constraints, but when you're face to face with human suffering in its most distilled form, it can't help but remind you of why you wanted to become a doctor in the first place.

I always tell the clinicians and residents I speak with that *we are all pain doctors*, whether we're specialists or primary care practitioners. Pain is an omnipresent symptom in medical practice; the majority of all office visits are instigated by pain. And yet, in its chronic form, pain remains one of the toughest conditions to treat, and can be impossible to cure. That's not the only reason many doctors dread their pain patients. These patients may often be suffering to the point of despair or distress, and present with symptoms that can be frustrating to treat. Many patients in pain have co-morbid psychiatric conditions that can make them even more difficult to manage. And there's the omnipresent concern that a few patients may be drug seeking or simulating pain for other benefits. We may also be concerned that the state medical board or the Drug Enforcement Administration (DEA) might be monitoring our prescribing habits to see if we're part of the diversion problem . . . not to mention our anxieties about side effects from medication, or adverse outcomes from procedures.

No wonder so much pain goes untreated or under-treated.

There is no debate among public health experts about the fact that pain is under-treated. Under-treatment of pain has been recognized as a public health crisis for decades. The consequences are often catastrophic for patients, in terms of suffering and disability, as well as for the healthcare costs we all share, since untreated and under-treated pain often lead to expensive utilization of resources.

But turning away from patients in pain simply isn't an option. Not if we are to meet our ethical responsibilities, and not if we care about our patients' well-being. If we are true to an age-old ethic of medicine, that we "cure when we can but treat suffering always," we must first and foremost respond to our patients' pain. And to do that, we need to cultivate the diverse skills that will enable us to engage effectively with our patients in pain.

Though we're all called upon to treat patients in pain, few of us were trained to respond to their special needs.

I have a personal theory about why so many doctors resist treating pain. It's not that they aren't compassionate people, or that they don't want to engage with difficult cases. *The problem is simply that most doctors aren't well prepared to manage pain.* And who enjoys doing something they aren't trained to do?

It's not surprising that most of us don't feel confident about our pain-management skills. Though we're all called upon to treat patients in pain, few of us were trained to respond to their special needs. Pain management is a very young discipline that's barely taught in medical school and residency, and Continuing Medical Education (CME) in pain management is currently only mandated in one state, California. Meanwhile, the science and technology of pain medicine is expanding at such a rapid rate that even specialists have a hard time keeping up with the literature about new concepts of pain transmission, medications, procedures, devices, and therapies.

The good news is that every clinician can become a more effective pain doctor—and it doesn't require going back to school or even earning CME credits. What it takes is a willingness to embrace a treatment paradigm that's at odds with much of our medical training. We've been trained to base our diagnoses and treatment choices on objective, verifiable symptoms—but pain is an *unprovable* and totally subjective symptom. We're taught to deal with our patients at an objective and rational distance. Yet treating pain requires getting close enough to a patient to peer inside his life, to discover the precious things that pain has taken away—and then figure out how to restore that loss. Simply put, we are called upon to heal what hurts, on both a physical and emotional level. The key to making this therapeutic connection with your patient is, in a word, communication.

That's why I've written this book. I'm convinced that if I can give you simple, practical tools for improving communication with your patients in pain, they will have better treatment outcomes, and you'll get more satisfaction from the care you give these patients. It's a win-win proposition.

Research bears this out: patients who feel that they have good rapport and communication with their doctors consistently report better treatment outcomes and higher levels of well-being and satisfaction. This body of research speaks to a central truth about treating pain: *simply acknowledging your patient's pain can have profound therapeutic effects.* Just knowing that a caregiver believes their pain exists and wants to help alleviate it makes it easier for patients to endure their pain. In fact, it actually reduces the intensity of their pain, which isn't surprising since pain is a totally subjective experience. Think back to when you were a young child and hurt yourself on the playground. A simple caring question from a parent or teacher—"Where does it hurt?—was often enough to salve the pain and dry your tears. People in pain feel isolated and are hypersensitive to being judged as faking or exaggerating their symptoms. They are starved for compassion.

But being compassionate and open to patients in pain doesn't come naturally. As human beings, we are hard-wired to avoid pain, whether our own or another's. Being a good pain doctor means resisting that instinct and squarely facing our patients' suffering. It means reaching out to them with compassion, asking personal and sometimes difficult questions—and then listening to their answers for clues about the source of their pain and suffering.

I've titled this book *Listening to Pain*, because listening to our patients is one of the best ways we can elicit useful diagnostic information in the murky world of pain and suffering. We're used to examining patients with our eyes and our hands. We know how to read and interpret their charts and their lab results. But it's a lot harder for us to tune into what our patients are telling us with their words and with their eyes, to use our inner ear to listen closely for clues to the source of our patient's suffering.

Here's an example, from my own practice, of the value of listening to pain . . .

I was asked by a hospice service to help with a difficult patient. All of the caregivers were utterly frustrated with this man whose prostate cancer had metastasized and who had a radiation-induced fistula in his buttock area. Normally, this situation would garner extreme sympathy, but this case went the exact opposite way. The man claimed to be in extreme pain and yet, for one reason or another, he rejected each and every medication that was offered. His doctors, nurses, and social workers were intensely frustrated. His family members didn't have the luxury of harboring strong negative feelings, but they were clearly at the end of their rope and were desperate for help.

He *was* being a tyrant at home. Even he was able to see that his refusal to accept treatment for his pain was hurting him and everyone around him. He was dying and in pain, and despite his behavior being atypical, he was entitled to have some bad days. I sat down with him and asked him to rate his pain on a scale of zero to 10, with

10 being the worst possible pain. "Ten," he said. I asked him why he didn't want to take the pain medications. He said that the side effects of constipation and sleepiness were unacceptable to him. He said "I can't believe we can send a man to the moon but you can't kill my pain without plugging me up or making me a zombie!" He repeatedly asked if we could just remove his painful leg or kill the nerves. I explained that surgical options, such as removing his leg, were most unlikely to take away his pain and that ongoing nerve blockade with a catheter was possible but posed significant risk in his situation because of the potential for infection. He didn't want to take that risk. He was basically putting everyone in a double bind. He was saying "Help me," but also "Don't help me because I won't accept risks or tolerate any side effects."

As I talked with him, it became clear to me that the problem wasn't simply nociception—I believed his pain was real, but his portrayal of sensations and intensities didn't sound like normal pain transmission. Often in these situations, this indicates that the pain signal has become distorted at some level. So instead of focusing on the pain and how we could treat it, I backed away from it and started asking him about his life and what exactly he was feeling. When I eventually came to the topic of his sleep, he told me he couldn't sleep well, even when he had used the sedating medications.

"Because of the pain?" I asked.

"No . . . I just can't turn these thoughts off in my mind," he said.

He went on to tell me of his ruminations about his disease, how his family will struggle without him, events in the future that he will miss, and many other profound but deeply agitating thoughts. He was afraid . . . afraid of dying, afraid about what would happen to his family, and concerned about all the logistical details of his household and finances. The fear interrupted his sleep, and his sleep deprivation exacerbated his fears *and* his pain. I also discussed his mood as well as what was so intolerable about the side effects he had from his previous pain medicines. In each case, he was clear that when he was even slightly sedated he wasn't able to do his routine activities. Thus, for him, life wasn't worth living. This meant working on his farm and doing things that helped his family with their daily lives. Unfortunately, he found himself in a vicious circle, having pain that slowed him down but didn't knock him out, or reducing the pain with medication but being too sedated to function. Either way, he became depressed. He couldn't sleep at night and became increasingly drowsy and irritable during the day because of sheer fatigue.

I decided to stop pushing pain medications on him. Instead, I prescribed a stimulant for the mornings to wake him up and keep him alert, which also acted as an antidepressant. I also prescribed a neuroleptic in the evenings to help reduce the impact of his fear on his sleep. It wasn't what his doctors were expecting, and they were frankly skeptical. Here was a dying hospice patient and I, the pain specialist, was not even offering anything resembling morphine or a typical analgesic regimen!

A week later his fistula was still a gaping wound and his prognosis was just as grim. But he now rated his pain as a *one* on the 10-point scale. He was able to relate to people, he had become much less belligerent and argumentative. He was back to being the person he once was, despite the presence of what was now a relatively low-grade pain.

My point here isn't that most chronic pain patients don't need pain medications. Far from it. This case was unusual in that respect. My point is that the key to solving this case, improving this patient's quality of life and reducing his pain was asking germane questions and *listening* carefully to his responses. I had to listen beyond his report of pain, to whatever was amplifying his sensations to such a horrid level, and then suggest a therapeutic course of treatment. As with most of my patients in pain, I had to shift my focus—and his—from treating his pain directly to improving what he clearly told me was most important to him—his general *functioning*. In this case, the key to reducing his pain and increasing his function was to *treat the pain magnifier*, which was a combination of sleep deprivation, fear, and depression.

This hospice patient represents the kind of patient many clinicians fear most: someone whose symptoms are unverifiable, who doesn't respond to treatments offered, who becomes a "black hole" of time and energy, and whose behavior radiates hostility and rejection. This is unfortunately how many chronic pain patients are perceived—and, indeed, such patients *are* difficult, often because they are frustrated, in pain, and they don't feel they've been listened to by a healthcare system that has become fragmented and focused on objective diagnoses that are provable with blood tests and radiological scans.

But a knee-jerk avoidance of patients in chronic pain by general practitioners amplifies the broader crisis of under-treated pain in this country. Because they can be difficult and noncompliant, it is tempting to move pain patients through the office rapidly, which sets up a feed-back loop of inadequate treatment, more pain, more visits, more hostility, and ever-diminishing satisfaction on the part of the clinician and patient.

Which brings us back to the power of listening. As clinicians we are trained to be scientists: we seek data, test results, x-rays, evidence from high-tech imaging equipment—anything that we can quantify and use as a basis for rational decision making. Pain, however, confronts us with a disconcerting opacity and symptoms that are influenced by such intangibles as a patient's beliefs, expectations, fears, and personality traits. These latter attributes are actually incredibly valuable sources of information to the clinician willing to mine them. But for the most part, clinicians have not been taught how to engage with chronic pain patients in a way that facilitates successful treatment outcomes.

A knee-jerk avoidance of patients in chronic pain by general practitioners amplifies the broader crisis of under-treated pain in this country.

I want this book to help fill the gap between the little you may have learned in medical school and the reality you confront at the bedside. I want to introduce you to effective strategies for communicating with and managing patients in chronic pain. This is *not* a book about specific treatments, diagnostic algorithms, or pharmacotherapy, all of which are useful and important but are presented elsewhere and tend to shift with emergence of new medications and procedures. My emphasis here is at a more fundamental level of establishing a therapeutic rapport with your patient. I have seen the value of these techniques in my own practice and in those of clinicians I have trained.

We need not be paralyzed by fear of difficult patients and complex cases, treatment risks, or regulatory oversight. We can be mindful of these concerns and still find a path that allows us to ease suffering and embody the altruistic aspirations that motivated our entry into a healing profession in the first place.

How to Use This Book. This is not a textbook. Rather, I encourage you to think of it as a personal tutorial from one clinician to another. In it, I've tried to offer the most specific and pragmatic guidance I can, distilled from my work as a pain medicine clinician, researcher, and educator. I've drawn on my own training in psychiatry, internal medicine, and anesthesiology. But mostly I've drawn from my direct experience with patients. Where useful as illustration, I've shared case studies, though I've changed any identifying details to protect the confidentiality of the patients.

I'm confident that the paradigm I'm offering you is a compassionate and effective strategy for treating chronic pain patients. It allows you to fulfill your ethical and professional obligations to attend to suffering, while also taking prudent steps to protect yourself against emotional burnout. And in my experience, adopting the principles and techniques outlined in this book will significantly improve the treatment outcomes of your patients.

Each chapter addresses a different aspect of improving pain management through better communication:

Chapter 1: Asking the Right Questions explains why taking a broad patient history is a crucial first step in assessing patients in pain. This history is the baseline for a clear document trail within the patient record. I'll tell you what questions you need to ask to elicit vital information about your patient, how to pose these questions, and how to hear and record the responses.

Chapter 2: Focusing on Function explains why focusing on numerical pain scales and subjective pain reduction can be less therapeutic than setting treatment goals and measuring treatment success through functional goals and outcomes. As the hospice patient anecdote illustrates, pain and pain tolerance are relative and subjective experiences, while functional outcomes are objective, measurable, and much more directly related to quality of life. Pain is destructive to the degree it deprives people of activities that give their life meaning and pleasure. This chapter focuses on linking pain management to the restoration of quality of life through targeting and improving function.

Chapter 3: Keeping Track of Treatment shows how documentation is an invaluable record of doctor-patient communication and a tool for risk assessment and management. Treating pain always involves *risk management.* All treatments—including doing nothing—involve some risk. The judgment call we need to make, as with any medical intervention, is always whether a potential risk outweighs a potential benefit. When someone is in pain, there is no risk-free treatment option, including non-treatment! The better we know our patients, the better we can make sound decisions regarding risk management.

Doctors tend to think of documentation as defensive medicine. While it is useful as a record of your rationale for whatever treatment regimen you and your patient elect, I also emphasize that you can improve your treatment outcome with clear documentation of the therapeutic relationship, including education on risks and benefits, informed consent, patient-selected functional goals, prescribing agreements, and follow-up evaluation and monitoring.

Chapter 4: Dealing with Difficult Patients gives you practical advice about how to use communication skills to manage different types of problem personalities and the conflicts they arouse in us as practitioners. I also touch on the difficult situations that arise with pain patients, such as what to do when a patient lies to you, fails a urine toxicology screen, or becomes aggressive and threatening.

Chapter 5: Clinician Survival. We're no good to our patients (and certainly not to our spouses and families) if we're burned out by the emotional demands of treating pain. In this chapter, I share my thoughts and techniques on how best to maintain perspective, recharge your batteries, and heal the psychological wounds we clinicians incur as the inevitable collateral damage of the war on pain.

Appendix: Resources for Pain Management. A huge amount of helpful information is now freely available via the Internet. I have selected what I consider the best such resources and have listed them in this section. On these sites, you can find useful documents for assessing, educating, and monitoring your patients. You can download copies of documents ranging from patient education handouts to sample pain treatment agreements, print them out and adapt them to the particular needs of your practice. The Internet is also a good place for patients to find support groups and other resources to overcome their sense of isolation, so I identify sites that you can be comfortable recommending to your patients. (Some sites are valuable for both patients *and* clinicians.)

There is no quiz at the end of this book. No CME credit. No score or accreditation. The true test of what you've learned is waiting for you in your office or clinic. Connecting with patients in pain and giving them the care they need and deserve is a career-long learning curve. Welcome to the journey!

Chapter 1
Asking the Right Questions

To hear about pain is to have doubt;
to experience pain is to have certainty.

— ELAINE SCARRY, *The Body in Pain:*
The Making and Unmaking of the World

I was called in to see a man who was recovering from recent abdominal surgery. When I walked into his room, the patient seemed to be oddly rigid and wasn't moving very much. As this was an academic teaching hospital, I was making rounds with a large group composed of fellows, residents, and students, and when we arrived in the room, the primary surgery team had just walked in to start their visit with this patient. I stepped back and allowed the surgery resident to conduct the interview and he started by asking the patient a question straight from the Joint Commission on Accreditation of Healthcare Organizations (JCAHO) protocol: "On a scale of zero to ten, with zero being no pain and ten being the worst pain you can imagine, how much pain are you in?" The man replied, "Zero." The treating team took that as reassuring information and moved on to the other questions and examinations relating to his post-operative course. And yet something was clearly wrong. Before leaving the room, I asked a simple question: "Does it hurt if you move or cough?"

"Hell yes!" the man said. It turned out that as long as he didn't move, he wasn't in pain . . . but he wasn't moving *because* moving was so painful. He figured anyone would be expected to have such pain after surgery and since no one had asked, he didn't mention it. He sure didn't want to be seen as a complainer or, worse yet, a drug-seeker. The man needed pain medication, but because he hadn't been asked the right question, the treating team arrived at the wrong conclusion and wasn't inclined to prescribe the needed medications.

Confronted with a patient in acute or chronic pain, a clinician today can select from an arsenal of diagnostic and evaluative tools. We can use magnetic resonance imaging (MRI), ultrasonography, and other imaging technologies to detect physiological abnormalities that might be causing pain. We can use electromyography, nerve conduction, and evoked potential studies to test the patency of specific nerve roots or pathways and try to rule in or out a myopathy, neuropathy, radiculopathy, or plexopathy. Reflex arcs can be evaluated, as can sensory abnormalities.

All of these can, at times, be helpful. But these tools can neither measure pain itself, nor prove or disprove the validity of a patient's claim that he or she is in pain. The old maxim "absence of evidence is not evidence of absence" applies with particular force when assessing pain. It seems inconceivable that the most common complaint brought to a clinician is an untestable hypothesis. But it's true. Once we get over this and accept that we can't prove or disprove pain or pain relief, we can get on with the business of relieving suffering and improving quality of life.

Various pain measurement scales exist and these, too, can be helpful—but they are not definitive. Unidimensional instruments such as the familiar numerical pain scale, the visual analog scale, and the "faces" pain rating scale can provide some degree of guidance about a patient's experience of pain, but all of these are completely subjective, open to wide variations between patients and within patients at different times. And again, no one can prove, disprove, or objectively measure pain itself. Multidimensional instruments, such as the McGill Pain Questionnaire or the Brief Pain Inventory provide a broader picture of a patient's experience, but are usually more cumbersome to administer, and in the end, suffer the same limitations as all other attempts to measure pain.

It seems inconceivable that the most common complaint brought to a clinician is an untestable hypothesis. But it's true.

We are left, therefore, with a simple, but accurate, maxim: "Pain is what a patient says it is." But as the prior anecdote illustrates, unless we ask the right questions, we may not get an accurate patient report on his or her pain.

Efforts to label pain as either "physical" or "psychological" usually serve no useful purpose. If you look at a functional MRI of the brain of a patient in pain, you'll see that the emotional centers of the brain—the limbic centers—are every bit as active as the sensory areas.

On a superficial level that might be surprising, because we tend to think of pain as a sensation. But if you look at it in its full human and psychosocial dimensions, pain is actually as much an emotional as a physical experience. There's also a striking overlap of the medical bags of psychopharmacologists and pain medicine practitioners. If you look at all the drug groups, you'll find that there is not a single drug group in psychiatry that isn't also used as an analgesic. Some pain patients fear this idea of pain as a mind/body phenomenon because they think we will conclude that their pain has no "physical" cause and it's "all in their head." I allay such fears by assuring patients that I take all pain seriously, regardless of negative findings from scans, tests, or lab results. You can't have pain without a head, so while I sympathize with patients who fear that I might think their pain is all in their head, I know that even if it is predominantly in their body, when there is pain, the mind and body are inextricably linked.

Anyone complaining of pain is suffering from something; it's our job to figure out what they're suffering from. The best way to begin assessing a patient's pain is to *ask* him or her about it and *listen* to what he or she tells us. That probably sounds self-evident, but in my experience, this is not what we usually do. All too often we get caught up in our attempt to quantify pain, pinpoint the cause of pain, categorize pain, and decide how best to treat pain. In the process, we fail to ask the right questions, we distance ourselves from our patients, we forget to focus on the whole person, and all too often we miss golden diagnostic clues that could lead to far more effective interventions.

Of course, many forces conspire to disconnect clinicians from their patients in chronic pain: lack of time, lack of training, concerns about the abuse potential of certain pain medications; the inherent subjectivity of the phenomena, and the sometimes difficult personalities of chronic pain patients—to name just a few. Unfortunately, if we succumb to these obstacles, we ourselves will end up suffering . . . sometimes more than our patients! We'll become frustrated, defensive, and ineffective clinicians. It doesn't need to be this way. I have found that taking three relatively simple steps at the very start of contact with a patient in pain can *reconnect* us with our patients, build an effective doctor/patient alliance, improve the efficacy of pain treatments, and increase personal satisfaction in our work:

Step 1: Slow Down.
Step 2: Focus On the Whole Patient, Not Just the Pain.
Step 3: Use Reflective Listening Skills.

Step 1: Slow Down

In some ways, my first suggestion—"slow down"—is the hardest to accomplish. Confronted with difficult patients or difficult cases, we tend to speed up as opposed to what is really needed—taking the extra time necessary to focus on the person and not just the pain. I know how busy clinicians are and how many people are dependent on us for help. But we don't do our patients or ourselves any favors by skimping on the details and assuming that we somehow know how our patients feel. The subjective and broad nature of pain demands that we take the time to listen.

The key here is to pause before seeing a patient and to consciously take the time to listen closely (including to others who might be present) as we proceed with a thorough history. As we talk with a patient, we need to ask questions not only about the pain (e.g., its location, intensity, duration), but also about the rest of a patient's life. To use a musical metaphor, we need to listen not just to the lyrics (the self evident parts of what the patient says) but to the music as well (the less obvious parts of verbal and non-verbal information about the rest of the patient's life). We need to be alert to subtle signs of trouble and take the time to ask follow-up questions.

Depression can dramatically alter pain perception—usually for the worse.

For example, a patient might casually mention that she's recently stopped driving. That can be an enormous issue since, for some, it can greatly decrease independence, limit social and work options, and significantly erode quality of life. These, in turn, can initiate a downward spiral of mood or cognition that can magnify the patient's pain perceptions. If it turns out that the patient lives in a condominium in a planned community serviced by shuttle buses, driving may not be a very important variable in her quality of life. But "I haven't been driving so much" could also mean that he or she lost his or her license because of drunk-driving arrests. You won't know unless you take the time to ask.

Step 2: Focus on the Whole Patient, Not Just the Pain

Although it might sound counter-intuitive, I often counsel my peers to take their focus *off* the pain and ask questions that allow them to get a fuller sense of the context in which the pain exists. I consider pain to be just one part of a matrix of symptoms related to suffering that must be assessed and treated as a whole. Pain is usually related to suffering that is interwoven with many unpleasant experiences, including fatigue, nausea, depression, anxiety, drowsiness, loss of appetite, insomnia, and a diminished sense of well-being. These are absolutely vital connections for a diagnostician—and if you miss them, you'll miss understanding the true dimensions of a patient's pain—*and* possible ways to alleviate that pain. For example, depression can dramatically alter pain perception—usually for the worse. If you don't ask direct questions related to mood, or pick up on the subtle signs that patients may offer in their answers that suggest neurovegetative deterioration, you may not recognize this significant factor in the experience of pain. Similarly, a host of life situations can affect pain, either directly (such as the use or abuse of licit or illicit drugs) or indirectly (such as high stress levels at work or home, or physical deconditioning caused by lack of exercise).

The story of a former patient of mine illustrates the point. Mark was a large, gruff man who came to me because the medications he'd been prescribed by other doctors hadn't worked to control his trigeminal neuralgia. After I finished with a pharmacological history, I asked him about his life. As a no-nonsense businessman, he was at first taken aback when I asked him about his family life, his job, and what gave him stress. But as his answers emerged, so did clues about what might be complicating his pain treatment.

Mark grew up in a tough neighborhood. His father was an alcoholic, his mother was depressed, and Mark was in and out of a dozen foster homes before he was 15. These experiences led to a pervasive anger against the world as a young adult and to a raging determination to both succeed and prove others wrong. He became a volatile workaholic—financially successful, but under tremendous emotional strain.

By the time he saw me, Mark's pain and the sedation caused by the original anti-convulsant medication had exacerbated his already short temper, which increased his stress at work. His facial seizures reduced him to whispering or mumbling, and eating was awkward and painful.

After listening closely to his stories, it was obvious that pain was now only part of his suffering. I realized that the only way to completely attack his pain was on both physical and emotional fronts. Trigeminal neuralgia is well known to have direct connections to emotions—in fact, laughing and crying can make it worse. I needed to find a way not only to quiet the hyperactive nerves, but to help him with his anger and stress while reversing the listlessness and slow thinking that accompanied the medication he was on.

I prescribed medications that have both analgesic and anti-anxiety effects. I also changed the anticonvulsant to one with a less sedating side-effect profile. Change didn't occur overnight. But with each small gain, Mark's trust in our approach grew. He was increasingly open to the possibility that the pain was being worsened by his state of mind. He accepted my recommendation to work with a cognitive behavioral psychologist who specialized in pain management—but not before I heard his deep concern about being labeled as having a mental illness, something he had experienced in his childhood as he moved through the foster care system. I tried to reframe the psychology of pain management using analogies from sports events, such as the Boston Marathon or the Tour de France. I presented the psychology of pain as essentially the same as the psychology of performance: developing internally powerful mechanisms for controlling our attention and how much sensation we actually feel. This was a much more acceptable model and, over time, he began to view learning new cognitive skills as hills to climb in his own personal marathon.

Clearly, Mark was beset with a physical disease, but his suffering was also intimately linked to his raging emotions. The key to his successful treatment outcome lay in the questions that ranged far from his specific pain experience, and in an approach that encompassed the totality of his situation, not just his pain.

Step 3: Use Reflective Listening Skills

Patients in chronic pain are frequently more emotional than they might be normally. They can also be more defensive, short-tempered, or even hostile. Under the circumstances, this isn't hard to understand. They're in pain, may have chronic disorders, and may have undergone previous treatments that didn't help or even made things worse. When conversing with these patients, I have found that the most effective approach is *reflective listening*. This means listening carefully and non-judgmentally to what your patients are saying, then reflecting it back to them in a slightly modified or reframed manner.

This is often easier said than done, because getting to the information we need is not always a trip the patient wants to take. These patients may have already been through many medical journeys, fraught with struggle and disappointments. Some may not be interested in or tolerant of a doctor delving into their personal lives. Our natural reaction when the patient is uncomfortable is to skim over the topic and leave vitally important areas unexamined. It is even worse when a patient makes a statement at odds with the evidence, or uses threatening or hostile language. Our natural reaction is to immediately defend ourselves, rebut the charges, or deny the underlying assumptions. Although understandable, this quickly creates a confrontational dynamic that can be difficult to reverse. It is much more effective to take a moment before speaking, and then to consciously try to simply restate what the patient just said. For example, if a patient says "Doctor, those pills you gave me don't work—I told you before that I need something stronger," you can reply "You're a little angry at me because you don't think the medications I prescribed are working for you." This way of responding offers a number of advantages because it:

- Is less likely to evoke or exacerbate patient defensiveness;
- Encourages the patient to keep talking and exploring the topic;
- Communicates respect and caring, and encourages a therapeutic alliance; and
- Offers an opportunity to clarify exactly what the patient means.

Although it can be particularly helpful when a patient is emotional, reflective listening is a useful tool in practically *all* patient interactions and can be used to follow up or probe answers to questions that you ask during a preliminary history-taking. For instance, this is a conversation where you might hear the initial response and move right along, but where you might do better to employ reflective listening:

Doctor: Has your chronic pain ever made you want to harm yourself or end your life?

Patient: No, not really.

Doctor: You're saying "not really," and I can take that in one or two ways. Either you haven't had suicidal thoughts, or you've had them, but they haven't alarmed you yet.

Patient: Well, I have thought about it, in a fantasy sort of way, but I don't think I would ever act on it.

Doctor: Have you ever tried to harm yourself before?

Patient: Yes . . .

As you can see, using reflective listening to go the extra round of dialogue unearthed an important detail that the patient had at first concealed. This also points out the hazards of asking two-part questions—such as do yourself harm or end your life. It's always better to break them into separate queries so you'll be confident you're getting complete answers.

The Importance of Taking a Comprehensive History

Listening to pain really means listening to the whole person. Getting the "story" means that you have to expand the typical list of questions asked during a history. No one size fits all patients or medical practice, so each clinician will need to evaluate the tools that work for him or her and perhaps even tailor the standard forms to his or her specifications.

I usually begin conversations with patients by asking about their pain, but then I move on to the broader contexts and impacts of that pain. Here are some of the points I try to cover in an initial evaluation:

■ Location of pain.
■ Character of pain. (Is it shooting or stinging? Does it increase at night or in the morning?)
■ How and when pain started.
■ Is pain continuous or intermittent?
■ Exacerbating and relieving factors—what makes it feel better or worse, including medication, rest, activity, stress, sleep, or hot showers?
■ Effect of stress on pain, as well as the source of stressors.
■ Effect of alcohol and other substances on pain.
■ Any sleep disturbances?
■ Any mood disturbances?
■ Any ongoing medical concerns?
■ How does pain affect functioning at school or work?
■ How does pain affect quality of life functions, such as relationships, sex, or recreation?
■ How do pain *treatments* affect important life functions, such as work, recreation, sex, or any other significant activity for the patient?
■ What does the patient expect from medications or other treatments in terms of analgesia or recovered function?

In the course of your conversations with patients, be alert to signs that they are minimizing their pain. Although it sounds counter-intuitive, some patients will fail to convey the true nature and severity of their pain and, thus, wind up undermining the effectiveness of their treatment. They may not want to distract the clinician from treating their primary disease, they may think they should just "suck it up" and endure their pain, they may think pain is simply inevitable with their illness, or they may not want to acknowledge that their disease is progressing. Some may worry that if they complain of pain, their doctor will see them as complainers, as demanding or weak—possibly even as addicts. Many people also under-report pain because they fear that pain medications will dull their mental abilities, lead to addiction, or have unmanageable side effects. And some patients fear that early pain control will preclude pain control later in the disease. They believe they'll become tolerant to their pain medications or that their doctors will lose interest in them if they have a failed medication trial. If you suspect a patient is minimizing pain, use reflective listening to probe for the concerns that may lie underneath the minimizing.

Doctor: How has your back pain been this past month?

Patient: It's not so bad . . . it doesn't really stop me from doing what I want.

Doctor: You say that it's not so bad and it's not interfering with what you want to do, but you've also reported problems sleeping because of the pain, and problems driving to work some mornings.

Patient: I guess it does keep me from getting a good night's sleep. The mornings are always worse if I don't sleep well the night before, which is most of the time, and I guess it does affect me at work, too.

The advantage of reflective listening is that it allows you to do your wondering and investigating in collaboration with your patient, rather than by yourself.

Once you've uncovered a patient's reasons for minimizing his or her pain, you can then directly address those concerns, correct mistaken notions, provide reassurance, and allay fears. When symptom minimization is very prominent, I have even asked patients directly: "Are you a stoic silent sufferer?" Being described as stoic is considered somewhat of a compliment to many patients and it's often a relief to the patient or to family members, who just needed permission to speak up about their pain.

Focusing on Function

I will have more to say in the next chapter about shifting your diagnostic and treatment paradigm from a focus on pain to a focus on the measurable impact of pain on the patient's function. Here I want to point out my inclusion of function-related questions in a pain history and emphasize their importance in structuring your early interactions with a patient. As I have said, pain is an untestable hypothesis—it isn't verifiable, it is highly subjective, and it can be influenced by a vast number of factors other than specific tissue or nerve damage. This means that tying your treatment goals to pain reduction alone is like trying to hit a moving target. Of course your patients are going to want to reduce their pain, however they may experience the sensation. But since you can't measure pain in the first place, you will have only the crudest means available to determine if you and the patient have achieved the goal of "pain reduction."

> *Tying your treatment goals to pain reduction alone is like trying to hit a moving target.*

I let patients know early on that I want to understand how their pain has impacted their daily lives. If, over the course of the day, their pain varies from a 4 to an 8 out of 10, I want to know what they can do when their pain is a 4 that they can't do when it is an 8. What meaningful activities are no longer possible and how were those activities lost over time? Once I can establish the level of functional losses related to pain, I can begin to envision possible goals for reclaiming lost functions.

I prefer to frame goals in terms of specific functional outcomes: return to playing golf, ability to make love again, returning to gainful employment or volunteer work, driving a car, attending a child's sporting event, or leaving the reclining chair in the living room and sleeping in their beds at night. These are measurable outcomes with direct significance and relevance to the patients. But in order to set such goals in the first place, I have to listen carefully to all patients and ask them specific questions about their functioning.

You must assess their current level of functioning in the important spheres of social, work-related, and interpersonal behaviors. You also need to find out what level of functioning the patient *wants or expects* to achieve from treatment. You can elicit useful information with questions, such as "Is there anything you can't do now that you could do previously?" and "What would you like to do that you can't do now?" Ultimately, these may prove to be much more important questions than those aimed simply at trying to target the nature and location of their pain. The answers to these questions will guide your treatment decisions, allow you and your patients to collaboratively establish objective treatment endpoints, and lay the groundwork for systematic and well-documented courses of action.

The Balancing Act of Compassion and Vigilance

All clinicians face the difficult challenge of conveying their empathy and compassion for a patient while at the same time remaining as objective as possible in their diagnosis and treatment decisions. This is doubly important when treating patients in chronic pain, who often feel misunderstood or distrusted by doctors. The inherently subjective nature of pain can lead patients to feel that nobody really understands their pain because it can't be verified with a test or a scan. As noted above, this can lead to defensiveness, suspicion, and hostility on the part of patients who in other contexts are perfectly reasonable, likeable people. We can go a long way toward reducing these negative feelings and behaviors by slowing down, widening our focus to include the whole person, asking the simple questions about a patient's life and passions, and then listening carefully to what we hear in response.

But it is clearly difficult to maintain a bond of empathy and support while simultaneously lifting every rock in a search for truth—including truths that the patient may not want to reveal. This conflict leads to a tension that is often palpable in the patient-clinician interaction. Your challenge is to maintain a tolerant, accepting and concerned tone in your conversation, while remaining persistent in your quest for the solid information you need to make prudent treatment decisions. When in doubt, suggest practical, nonjudgmental solutions to conflicting information.

Doctor: Your wife tells me you barely get out of your lounge chair during the middle of the day, yet you report that you're doing your physical therapy every afternoon, as we agreed you would.

Patient: She's at work all day, so how would she know what I'm doing from noon till three? She treats me like an invalid, but I'm not as helpless as she thinks.

Doctor: What I'm hearing you say is that you're a lot more functional than your wife thinks you are. While it's often difficult for others to understand what our lives are like, it can also be hard to be objective observers of ourselves. I have a suggestion. Why don't you keep a diary between now and your next appointment? Many of my patients have found that writing down their daily activity levels makes it a lot easier to keep track of what they actually did each day. Then we'll review it together and see if we can get a clearer picture of what your daily routine looks like.

The more questions you ask, and the more consistently you ask them over the course of long-term treatment, the more likely you are to gain insight into your patient's progress. In the pain management business, we must always be vigilant but rarely judgmental. You need to believe in your patients and involve them as much as possible in the decision-making process. You should be supportive and honest, neither promising too much nor removing all hope. By avoiding confrontation and fostering a spirit of alliance, we can be compassionate *and* highly effective healthcare providers.

Chapter 2
Focusing on Function

The good physician treats the disease; the great physician treats the patient who has the disease.
— WILLIAM OSLER, Physician, 1849-1919

In 1928 a baby girl was born in Montreal to a clinician and his wife. The delivery was normal, and the little girl appeared healthy in every way. But as the months passed, her parents began to feel that there was something odd about the child. As the years wore on, the startling truth of the girl's condition became distressingly obvious: she felt no pain. She never had a headache. She never had a toothache, a stomachache, an earache, or any discomfort from cuts or bruises.

Although at first glance, an inability to feel pain sounds highly attractive, the girl's parents knew better: her condition was actually life-threatening. This fact was made clear one winter's day. Alone in her room, the girl heard some children playing in the snowy street outside. She went to her window and, in order to see more clearly, knelt on a hot radiator. Minutes passed before she grew tired of watching the street scene. Then she got off the radiator and walked away, oblivious to the severe burns on both her legs.

Her parents discovered the burns and immediately rushed her to the hospital where she underwent extensive skin grafts to repair the damage.

The girl was formally evaluated when she was 20 years old and, as "Miss C" she became the first case of hereditary sensory and autonomic neuropathy reported in the medical literature. [*] By then, her hands, legs, and feet were scarred from cuts, bites, burns, scratches, and frostbite. In addition, her tongue was deformed from severe biting—some intentional during childhood, some unintentional in later years from normal accidents during eating which went unnoticed. She had also been hospitalized repeatedly for serious bacterial infections of her joints.

Thanks to antibiotics, Miss C survived those infections, had a relatively normal upbringing, and graduated from college. She was described in the published report as "very capable and cooperative and displaying remarkable initiative" in her work as an assistant in a university psychology department. But her health problems escalated. Her bones and joints began to break down and deform from the years of unintentional punishment. She could no longer walk, and the infections became more severe. In 1957, Miss C. was hospitalized again because of massive bacterial infections. The most powerful antibiotics of the day were ineffective. A month later, at the age of 29, Miss C was dead.

* McMurray G.A. Experimental Study of a Case of Insensitivity to Pain. *Archives of Neurology and Psychiatry*, 1950;64:650-657.

The Myth of Zero Pain

Miss C's tragic story drives home a point often lost in clinical settings: no healthy person goes through life pain-free. We all live with a wide range of low-grade pains, from muscle stiffness, cuts, bruises, headaches, sore limbs . . . you name it. In fact, some people live and function well with even moderate pain such as from arthritis or old injuries. While pain thresholds are similar from person to person, pain tolerance varies greatly among individuals, among different cultures, and in different environments. It's often remarked upon that women in labor can have extremely high pain tolerance, probably caused by a combination of hormonal release and an understanding that they are experiencing "purposeful pain."

On a parallel plane, we all live with varying degrees of psychic and emotional pain. Emotions like sadness, fear, anxiety, and anger, as well as childhood memories, all contribute to the landscape of pain. And each of us has a different tolerance for emotional pain, a different tipping point at which anguish makes us dysfunctional, when we become too depressed or dis-

> *We all live with varying degrees of psychic and emotional pain.*

traught to work or play or even take care of ourselves. Measuring the intensity of emotional pain is as subjective and elusive as quantifying physical pain. Measuring the amount of functional loss caused by pain, however, is an objective and quantifiable calculation.

The traditional zero-to-10 pain scale that we use so often in a clinic inadvertently implies that the ideal condition is "zero pain." It becomes all too easy, then, for doctors and patients to assume that the goal of pain treatment is the elimination of pain. As I hope to demonstrate in this chapter, this approach is fraught with pitfalls. Even the more modest goal of pain *reduction* misses the essential point: *the direct sensation associated with pain is not the only important variable and may not be the most important feature of the overall presentation of pain.* The real key to understanding pain and formulating an effective treatment plan is to look beyond the pain sensations to how those sensations are eroding a patient's quality of life. Specifically, how is the patient's pain affecting his or her *functioning* in daily life?

I suggest that you broaden your attention beyond the pain signals themselves to include a careful evaluation of the *effects* those signals are having on patient functioning. You can then use this knowledge to create a solid foundation for treatment decisions and patient management. Shifting from an analgesic to a function-based paradigm offers the following tangible advantages:

- Objective and verifiable treatment goals and outcomes, as opposed to untestable and subjective ones.
- Respect for individual differences among patients, both in terms of pain tolerance and functional goals.
- A more quantifiable basis for making risk/benefit decisions about pain-treatment options.

- A defensible rationale for prescribing decisions (including decisions to *terminate* a drug regimen).

Most important, *a function-based treatment strategy is much more likely to increase your patient's function and improve his or her quality of life.*

This is a paradigm shift for many clinicians because we traditionally focus almost exclusively on a patient's pain—and we believe that our job is to get rid of that pain. But simply reducing a patient's pain score from, say, a 9 to a 3 is only one piece of a much larger puzzle. And, to the surprise of many, it may not be the most important piece. Here's an example.

One of my patients was Mike, a 38-year-old construction worker. He sustained some lumbar disc injury from a work-related lifting injury and underwent laminectomy and fusion surgery. Unfortunately, the expected bone regrowth didn't occur and the fusion surgery had to be repeated. This fusion appeared to work, but he continued to be in pain. Several nerve-block procedures failed to bring relief.

When Mike first came to me he had been housebound for many months. His family was scraping by on his disability insurance payments, he lacked energy, slept in his reclining lounge chair, and was often irritable and short-tempered with his wife and children. He reported that the Vicodin he was prescribed both times after his surgeries had worked well at controlling his pain. But his wife, who accompanied him to our meeting, mentioned that he had used opioids as party drugs in college and that he tried to get as much Vicodin as he could following his surgeries.

This is not an atypical situation and vividly illustrates how clinical decision-making is usually a matter of balancing potential risks against potential benefits. It would be hard to deny Mike opioid medications (if they were the only treatment left for his pain) solely because he had an alleged history of liking these drugs and using them recreationally many years ago. But the real decision to be made here wasn't about opioids or Mike's potential for addiction. It was about Mike's functioning—or lack thereof—and about finding a strategy that would improve his activity level, restore his self-esteem, and rebuild his quality of life.

As I do with all my patients, I asked Mike a simple question: "What is it that you're going to do on this medicine that you can't do now?" At first he wasn't sure. "I don't know," he said. "I just want to feel better, that's all."

This might sound like a satisfactory response. But it's not. As I've said before, pain is an untestable hypothesis. Making the subjective report of "feeling better" our primary treatment outcome, means our outcome is untestable since we have no way, aside from the patient's testimony, to confirm that we achieved our goal. That can put the clinician at a real disadvantage. Relying solely on the patient's report means that you might miss evidence that the medication is not, in fact, effective, or is producing side-effects that are actually *reducing* quality of life despite the patient's claims to the contrary.

Simply "feeling better" may be an acceptable result of treatment. But feeling better without improving one's function, in at least in some aspects of life, is unacceptable. Chronic pain diverts a patient's attention from his or her normal life and slowly erodes his or her physical and emotional well-being. Relieving pain should lead to regaining the collateral losses associated with that pain—regaining lost function, in other words. If it does not, I believe the treatment should be deemed a failure, and another approach devised.

I explained all of this to Mike, as well as the related information that all medications have risks. And with opioids, it's not just the risk of abuse and addiction, it's the risk of sedation, sweating, constipation, itching—a host of possible side effects. The only way such a risk is acceptable is if the potential benefit is even greater—and the benefit has to be tangible and verifiable. I asked him to think about what components of life he has lost because of his injury and subsequent pain and what components he hopes to regain by using the medication.

"Well, I'd love to play rugby again," he said after a moment.

It was an understandable goal, and one that could be verified by others. But it was also unrealistically ambitious—particularly because he hadn't played since well before his back injury.

We talked some more and in the end we agreed on a set of realistic functional goals: he would aim to sleep in his bed again, attend a function at his son's elementary

school, enroll in a pain education class, and begin a program of gentle but long term physical therapy. As part of
this contract—which we developed together in writing—
we agreed that he would bring records from his class and
physical therapy sessions and his wife would confirm his
progress in the other areas and would attend a follow-up
meeting in a month.

In addition to this conversation, I gave Mike and his
wife some educational materials about the medications he
would be using, and an informed consent form that clearly laid out both the potential risks of the medications as
well as his responsibilities as a patient. Such education and
communication efforts in the earliest phases of treatment
are absolutely critical for laying a firm foundation for later
decisions. You have to communicate clearly, explain your
expectations and treatment goals, and educate the patient
as much as possible about the medication and how to use
it. Much of this work can be done by others on your staff,
or even through materials presented before or after you
see the patient.

Four weeks later Mike and his wife came in for a follow-up meeting. He had titrated up his opioid dose as
prescribed (I always follow the "start low, go slow" philos-
ophy to minimize side effects). Mike was smiling, but he
looked a little sleepy.

"The medication is really working doc," Mike said.
"My pain's gone from an 8 to a 2 most of the time."

Mike insisted that he was feeling better. And many
clinicians might stop right there because, after all, if the

patient says they're better, who are we to argue? But in this case, the best interest of my patient was a treatment outcome that addressed the root of his medical problem, reversed dysfunction, and promoted true health and wellness rather than simply a medicated facade of well-being.

As I began asking specific questions about the functional goals we had laid out earlier, it became clear that Mike had not actually made progress. He was still sleeping in the lounge chair, for example. He missed the school science fair he had said he'd attend. He hadn't attended the educational sessions and had only seen the physical therapist once. He also wasn't sleeping well . . . even though he felt sleepy most of the time. His wife reported that he was sleepy all the time and slept in short blocks of two to three hours, both at night and during the day. Apparently, Mike spent most of his waking time watching television.

Many clinicians might see in this pattern of behavior signs of an addiction. Mike was clearly using the drug without obtaining any real functional benefit. Perhaps he was enjoying the medication too much, but that was hard to determine. I believe clinicians must be very careful with the label "addict." I draw a distinction between a "chemical coper" and an addict. Many people are "chemical copers" either with legal or illegal drugs. They use drugs to cope with life and remain relatively healthy and functional despite, perhaps, being chemically dependent on a drug. Addicts, on the other hand, have a disease that impairs their ability to control or modulate their use of a drug that is causing them dysfunction. They also continue to crave and use the drug *despite* the dysfunction. For an addict, enough is never enough.

Mike seemed to be living somewhere between these two states—but I didn't need to put him in one box or the other because one thing was blatantly clear: he wasn't any better functionally. And, despite his own testimony, it was clear that the sedation he was experiencing was interfering with his ability to make progress toward our agreed-upon goals. The medications I prescribed were simply not working. After several trials with other opioids and approaches, I had to tell him, "Look, I'm sorry, but this is not an acceptable outcome for me and I can't allow your life to further erode. The opioids are not improving your condition like you think they are, and we have to transition off of them and try other approaches."

Addicts have a disease that impairs their ability to control or modulate their use of a drug that is causing them dysfunction.

I explained that it might be possible to find a clinician willing to keep giving him opioids and that seeking other opinions would in no way change what I had to do next or what I would be willing to do for him in the future. I then began the process of slowly tapering down and discontinuing his opioid regimen. I was also careful to educate Mike and his wife about withdrawal symptoms, how to deal with these symptoms if any arose and, most important, how tapering slowly and consistently should effectively avoid any adverse effects.

Taking this tack with pain patients—insisting that they discontinue opioids if they're not increasing their function—makes many clinicians uneasy. But it is exactly the same situation we face in many other realms of medicine. For example, if a diabetic has a life threatening case of vasculitis, corticosteroids may effectively ease their symptoms. But corticosteroids worsen glucose control. How do you handle the diabetic who argues that the only time he or she feels normal or even pain free is when he or she is on corticosteroids? What do you do when this patient asks for chronic dosing of corticosteroids, because they are the only way the patient can live without pain? Because of the severe toxicity of chronic corticosteroids in a diabetic, few of us would accommodate such a request. Most would clearly recognize that the benefits do not outweigh the risks. So as a doctor you are forced to say, "I'm sorry, but you can't have this medication even though it feels good because it's going to harm you in the long run." A patient who continues using an opioid medication, but whose quality of life is either unchanged or actually worse, is in the same boat—and our response, as clinicians, must be the same: "You can do better."

In Mike's case, we tried other opioids, because some are better tolerated than others in certain individuals. Determining which patient will do well on one drug but not the other is usually impossible to know in advance—idiosyncratic responses are the norm. So, we gave a few other opioids a try, in each case choosing long-acting formulations that avoided the roller coaster ups and downs of the short acting forms. After another month or so, little had changed and in fact, the sedation he had with the first opioid was replicated with those that followed. His functioning had declined, at least in part because of chronic sedation.

Looking at the big picture of Mike's life suggested to me that opioids, as a class, simply weren't going to be an effective route to improving his quality of life and possibly would cause harm. As we continued to talk, Mike began opening up about his feelings. He said he lay awake at night, worrying about how he would support his family and regretting the things he could no longer do. He also admitted that he was angry and felt humiliated at being so disabled. I realized that this man had lost much of his will to live and wanted, instead, to lose himself in an opioid fog.

A Different Approach

I suggested a new strategy. I reviewed with Mike and his wife the functional goals we had agreed upon in the first meeting, and I explained the reasons for using these as our guideposts rather than whether or not Mike "felt better." I focused on improving Mike's sleep/wake cycle, since fractured sleep, alone, can disrupt mood, sap motivation, erode energy levels, and magnify pain. In place of the opioids, I prescribed a non-addicting stimulant in the morning and a sedating medication that treated Mike's fear and anxiety for the evening. And for the short run, we focused on two related goals: having him sleep at night and not during the day, and sleeping in his bed instead of the recliner. This is an important part of setting functional goals: setting realistic, achievable goals and moving slowly, one step at a time. People want to take a pill and be better in a week. In the case of chronic illness marked by slow and longstanding deconditioning, recovery requires reconditioning that usually takes an equivalent period of time. I tell patients that this is a marathon, not a sprint. And I consistently find that if a patient can achieve one goal, their motivation and attitude improves, making the next goal that much easier to achieve. As with other life pursuits, gradual progress toward functional goals proves the truth of the adage, "The key to success is success."

Of course, I didn't ignore Mike's pain. He was concerned about my abandoning him to his pain, and he was frankly skeptical that he could make any progress without the opioids. He could still use non-opioid pain medications—and I encouraged him to do so as long as he didn't exceed the daily limits I suggested. But focusing on pain reduction did not get us where we needed to be and it was no longer my primary focus. We all needed Mike to concentrate on improving functioning in his daily life.

Two weeks later I called to follow up. It had not been easy for Mike to taper off of the opioids; he was even more cranky around the house and seemed, at first, more resistant than ever to making progress. But after a few weeks, he said he just got tired of lying around. He began to get up from his chair and take a few steps. Then he would sit down again. A week later, he slept in his bed for the first time in months. He said the intensity of his pain had increased, but he was able to taper off of his medications and get moving by using some of the techniques he had learned from the pain psychologist.

Two weeks later, Mike had attended two meetings of a chronic pain support group, and his wife reported that he had been regularly attending physical therapy. It was very good progress. And now I felt comfortable enough to prescribe moderate dosages of other analgesics. I was very clear with Mike that finding the right ones would be a trial and error experiment, and that if he sank back into his previous behavior patterns, we would discontinue the medication. But if the medication helped him achieve his functional goals, and if he adhered to the regimen without dose escalation, we could consider the medication effective. He clearly understood now that it wasn't in his interest to take anything—prescribed nor not—that didn't directly help him achieve his goals.

Four weeks later Mike and his wife came in for a visit. I could see the positive change on Mike's face, even before he spoke. He looked relaxed and alert. His pain was not gone; he said it varied from about a 3 to a 5 (out of 10) from day to day. But he could live with that. Indeed, he *was* truly living for the first time since his initial surgeries. He was moving around, making slow but steady progress in physical therapy, and becoming socially active. He was benefiting from a positive feedback loop I have observed in other patients: a relatively minor reduction in pain can lead to great improvements in function, which, in turn, can further reduce the importance of pain in their lives, which further increases function.

In my experience, a 20-percent reduction in a pain score (i.e., two points on the standard pain scale) is a perfectly acceptable goal and one that can produce significant benefits for a patient. The illustration below shows how seemingly modest reductions in pain can translate into dramatic functional improvement. If you tell your patient that you're going to reduce their pain by 20 percent, they may feel your analgesic goals are too modest. But if instead you frame your treatment outcome in terms of reclaimed functions lost to those two points on the pain scale, you're much more likely to motivate your patient.

Activities Impaired by *Increasing* Pain Severity*					
					Relate
				Walk	Walk
			Sleep	Sleep	Sleep
		Active	Active	Active	Active
		Mood	Mood	Mood	Mood
	Work	Work	Work	Work	Work
Enjoy	Enjoy	Enjoy	Enjoy	Enjoy	Enjoy
3	4	5	6	7	8
>>>>>>>>>>>> Worst Pain Rating >>>>>>>>>>>>					

* Assessed in cancer pain patients
Source: Cleeland CS, Ryan KM, *Ann Acad Med Singapore.* 1994;23:129-138.

Mind you, I don't recommend making reductions in pain scores the primary focus of your treatment goals for all of the reasons I've just explored. The pain score may be more important to patients than to clinicians. A pain score allows patients to economically communicate with their healthcare providers and can provide them with a quantitative yardstick with which to measure their sensations. But pain is so subjective that a single pain score provides only the crudest guide for a clinician. At best, pain scores can help detect changes from some baseline over time.

Monitoring Functional Changes

Obviously, if you are going to set functional goals for a patient (rather than basing treatment on whether or not the patient "feels better"), you need a way to know if goals have been met. This does *not* mean you have to become a private investigator to check up on each patient. Your goal is to work with a patient to agree on realistic goals with ways to verify their achievement of their goals. The responsibility of obtaining the "hard data" lies with the *patient*. At the top of the next page are examples of some functional goals I have set with patients and ways we found to confirm that the goals are achieved.

For functional goals in which the validation comes from a report from a spouse, partner, or friend, I ask that this person accompany the patient on follow-up visits or send me a signed note. Of course, no validation scheme is 100-percent foolproof—if somebody really wants to fool

Functional Goal	Evidence
Begin physical therapy	Letter from therapist
Sleeping in bed as opposed to lounge chair	Report by spouse or friend
Participation in pain support group	Letter from group leader
Walk around the block	Pedometer recordings
Walk without crutches	Report by spouse or friend
Resume sexual relations	Report by partner
Return to work	Pay stubs from employer
Daily exercise	Gym membership or spousal report

me, they'll find a way. But I believe that if you are willing to stick with the relationship for a moderate amount of time, dysfunctional patients usually declare themselves. They rarely are able to keep up a charade of documenting functional improvement when there is none. If a patient is really looking for access to an abusable prescription drug, they will probably leave when they see a function-based approach, and particularly when they are asked for evidence of adherence.

But the purpose of validating treatment goals is *not* to prevent abuse of prescription drugs, though it may certainly have that effect. The real purpose of putting "teeth" into an agreement on functional goals is to motivate patients to achieve their goals and to provide you with the information you need to determine if a given course of treatment is really working or not.

Functional goal-setting isn't a one-time event. Over a long-term therapeutic treatment course, you need to continually move the functional goalposts—in collaboration with your patient. This means that at each follow-up visit, you and your patients review their progress—or lack of progress—toward the agreed-upon goals. Much like a sports coach, if a patient has achieved a goal or set of goals, you want to calibrate those goals to motivate the patient to move up to the next level. For instance, if a patient, after three months of incremental improvement, has been able to return to swimming laps once a week, you might set a goal of swimming three times a week. Conversely, if you've set too ambitious a goal and your patient is becoming discouraged by the lack of progress, you can bring the goal down a notch.

"Universal Precautions" in Pain Management

When I'm setting up functional treatment goals with patients, they occasionally balk at my request for verification. "Don't you trust me doctor?" they ask.

I explain to them that in matters of patient-clinician partnerships, I cleave to the same Russian proverb that Ronald Reagan liked to quote: Trust, but verify. If the patient and I can agree on a verification protocol, then the issue of "trust" becomes moot. For example, doctors do not simply rely on the report of their diabetic patients that they have been diligent in testing their blood for high blood sugar. All such patients are asked to undergo a laboratory blood test to confirm and monitor their blood sugar levels over the past several months. In the same way, I explain, *all* my chronic pain patients are asked to provide some kind of evidence that they are making progress toward their functional goals as well as evidence that they are not being adversely affected by the treatment.

This approach is consistent with a relatively new paradigm in the field of chronic pain that has been called "universal precautions"—a term borrowed from the field of infectious diseases. The term "universal precautions in pain medicine" refers to a standardized approach to the assessment and ongoing management of *all* chronic pain patients. Just as it is impossible to predict if a patient (or their body fluids) will harbor an infectious agent, it's impossible to predict with any degree of certainty which pain patients will become problematic users of prescription medications.

> *It's impossible to predict with any degree of certainty which pain patients will become problematic users of prescription medications.*

Even when the medications being prescribed are not abusable, the issue of patient adherence to both medication and other therapeutic regimens is paramount. By applying uniform and standardized assessment and management approaches to *all* patients, we can reduce stigma, improve patient care, and contain overall risk. This means, among other things, not relying on "trust" when it comes to monitoring functional treatment outcomes. "Trust" in this case, may even be a cop-out for a clinician who doesn't want to bother with the task of monitoring adherence—whether to a medication or a treatment goal. The core issue here is simple transparency. As long as a system of verification doesn't stigmatize or discriminate against certain groups of patients, it takes the tension out of the therapeutic relationship of relying exclusively on patient reports.

In this chapter I've presented a new treatment paradigm that can liberate you from the often murky terrain of chronic pain management. In place of unverifiable and subjective pain symptoms, you can base your assessment and treatment plan on objectively recordable goals and outcomes. Instead of relying exclusively on patient reports and all the difficulties inherent in that model, you can collaborate with your patients to set clear and objective goals and a system for verifying progress toward them. Best of all, a function-based strategy lets you focus your treatment plan on tangible behaviors. This function-based strategy shifts the focus away from incalculable assessments of "how bad I feel" to a stepwise progression of quantifiable gains and improvements in quality of life.

You don't need expensive interventions or high-tech diagnostics to embark on a function-based treatment plan. All you need is a pen, paper, and the information you've gleaned from an in-depth conversation with your patient. As you integrate this approach into your practice, keep these principles in mind:

- Elimination of all pain (i.e., "zero" pain) is neither possible nor desirable.
- A patient's pain score is just one of many variables related to his or her overall status and potential for recovery.
- Treatment goals should *not* be set primarily in the form of changes in pain scores.
- Pain score reductions of as little as 20 percent can be extremely significant in terms of reclaimed function.
- Functional goals should be set collaboratively between patient and doctor, be realistic and achievable, be meaningful to the patient, and be verifiable.
- Functional goals should be revisited and recalibrated at regular intervals by both doctor and patient.
- Because patients vary in the functions they desire in life, each patient will have a unique set of functional treatment endpoints.

Chapter 3
Keeping Track of Treatment

Science is organized knowledge.
Wisdom is organized life.
— IMMANUEL KANT

In the first two chapters I've laid the groundwork for a pain-management paradigm based on:

■ Communication,

■ Compassion,

■ Detailed patient history to yield a three-dimensional profile of the "whole" patient, and

■ Functional treatment outcomes.

Now I want to show you how to integrate this approach into the real-world environment of your practice. We work in a wide range of environments, but there is one common denominator in our management of patients in pain—*the need to clearly document treatment.*

I'll show you that keeping a clear document trail can help make your practice *easier, more efficacious,* and more *personally rewarding.*

Why Documentation is a Doctor's (and Patient's) Best Friend

You might be wondering what clear documentation has to do with improved doctor-patient communication. In fact, they're both closely connected to the goal of building some objective and concrete data points into pain management. The chief value of open and clear communication between you and your patient is that such communication allows you to elicit important assessment information, as well as collaborate productively with your patient in establishing a treatment regimen.

Creating and maintaining a thorough written record is in the patient's *best interest.*

Documentation is the concrete record of your ongoing communication with your patient. It's what makes that communication both transparent and enduring. While documentation is important in the management of any patient, it's particularly valuable in pain management because of all the moving parts—physical, emotional, and psychological—involved in the treatment relationship.

Not only is clear, consistent, and detailed documentation part of "best practices," is it also the *only* way you will be able to reliably and legitimately assess the effectiveness of the treatment regimen. Of course, documentation is also valuable to you as a record of your rationale for a particular treatment regimen, but the point here is that creating and maintaining a thorough written record is in the *patient's* best interest. Given the impossibility of remembering the details of all your patients, the written record will be the only way you'll be able to spot trends over time, whether they be goals for or progress toward functional outcomes, severity of side effects, or slow changes in patient demeanor or affect. In addition, if you eventually need to refer your patient to a specialist, this documentation will enable continuity of care for your patient.

Everybody wins when your clinical behavior and decision making is as *transparent* as possible. This means that not only have you documented your care, but you have also adequately communicated your decision-making process, and most particularly, *why* your patient is taking medical risks. Remember that medicine hinges on risk/benefit assessment. Both treating and *not* treating involve risks, hence we cannot avoid being risk managers. Transparent documentation is the part of risk management where we record as clearly as possible how the risk/benefit analysis played out for a particular patient— it's the rationale for why we did or did not take action, and which treatment we and our patient chose.

A wide range of computerized systems are now available that offer tremendous advantages for the acquisition, storage, integration, and presentation of medical information. Most offer advantages that will benefit both the patients (because their information is kept up-to-date) and clinicians (because information relevant to prescribing or treatment is instantly available).

However, clear documentation is not dependent on com-puterization or electronic record-keeping; it's dependent on your commitment to keeping a clear written record in a system-atic fashion. Paper and pen or the dictated word work just fine.

Elements of Effective Documentation

Regardless of the logistical systems used to document your clinical decisions, detailed, readily available, and transparent documentation within the patient medical record should cover the following areas:

- Medical history and physical examination;
- Diagnostic, therapeutic, and laboratory results;
- Evaluations and consultations;
- Treatment objectives;
- Discussion of treatment risks and benefits;
- Informed consent;
- Treatments;
- Medications (including date, type, dosage, and quantity prescribed);
- Instructions and agreements; and
- Periodic reviews of patient behaviors, side effects, and functional outcomes.

There are four basic activities you want to be sure to document well:

1. Assessment
2. Education
3. Treatment Agreements
4. Monitoring

1. Assessment

Assessment should be based on a detailed patient history (which may be self-administered), medical records, physical examination, and a thorough face-to-face interview and discussion. By "assessment" I mean not only an accurate evaluation of the patient's medical condition and possible etiologies, but also a profile of all of the other potentially relevant parts of the patient's life, including mental or emotional factors (e.g., mood disturbances, cognitive impairment, active substance abuse), lifestyle considerations (e.g., lack of in-home support, family stressors, recent loss), and functional losses.

Assessing Risk and Benefit. As clinicians, we routinely weigh the potential risks and benefits of any treatment plan. It's what we do, and it's the reason why no treatment algorithm or computer program can replace a clinician's judgment and knowledge of his or her patients. It's also the reason I encourage you to take a comprehensive history and fill in any blanks with further conversation and questioning. If you invest the necessary time up front to obtain complete and reliable information, you will be in a far better position to make appropriate risk-benefit assessments on behalf of your patients.

It may seem self evident that we should maintain a balanced perspective on risk, always weighing the potential benefit of a treatment against its risks. But in the face of the complexity of pain, it's easy to become overwhelmed by the fear of risk in pain management and decide that the least risky course is to *not* treat the pain.

When someone is in pain, doing nothing (or under-treating) can be the riskiest decision of all.

The risks of non-treatment can be dire when it comes to pain. Indeed, pain can be fatal if left untreated. An overstatement? Hardly. Consider the case of a 76-year-old woman who comes into an emergency room with rib fractures. Adequately treating her pain is not just a matter of relieving her suffering: inadequate lung inflation and efforts to suppress coughing because of pain will increase her risk of life-threatening pneumonia.

While most cases aren't this dramatic, ongoing pain erodes quality of life and slowly deconditions a person's physical *and* emotional well being. Both directly (through abnormal activation of stress hormones) and indirectly (for instance by inducing inactivity, insomnia, anxiety, or depression), pain leaves sufferers vulnerable. Chronic pain also undermines the management of any pre-existing chronic condition (such as diabetes or cardiovascular disease) and psychiatric conditions (such as anxiety or depressive disorders).

When you look at the complete landscape of pain and its collateral damage, you'll see that pain offers us no risk-free option, including doing nothing. Not treating pain, in other words, is not a "safe" option for a patient. And *the risk of non-treatment* must always be factored into a decision about any pain treatment. Although this may seem obvious, clinicians face patients in pain each day and choose what they perceive as the lesser of evils: less treatment and less "risk."

Screening Patients at High Risk for Addiction or Abuse is Part of Risk Assessment. When considering long-term opioid use for pain management, you must assess your patient's potential and risk for abusing these drugs. Exactly who to suspect and when to be proactive in investigating risk factors is an area of great debate and investigation among specialists in pain and addiction medicine. From my review of the literature, there are no convincing data to support a strategy of focusing on any specific population—which means we all must be vigilant with anyone for whom we might consider prescribing controlled substances.

When you do uncover positive findings, be careful to avoid the tendency to over-react. Keep in mind that there are few absolute red lights from a screening session. Chronic pain is rarely an emergency, despite how a certain case may make you feel, and there is almost always time to deliberate or review more information before proceeding. Investigating risk of drug abuse is uncomfort-

Investigating risk of drug abuse is uncomfortable ground for most clinicians.

able ground for most clinicians, who may be reluctant to raise such sensitive personal issues with patients or risk being perceived as invading their privacy. It can also lead to conflict and clinician-patient tension. Resist the temptation to feel bad for maintaining your vigilance about risks of abuse; we are *obligated* to remain vigilant. The key is being clear that suspicions are not the same as judgments!

Several tools for assessing risk of addiction have been developed. CAGE is a classic tool developed for alcohol abuse that can easily be modified for any abusable drug. This brief questionnaire asks whether a patient has ever:

C: Wanted or needed to **C**ut down on drinking or drug use?

A: Been **A**nnoyed or **A**ngered by others complaining about his or her drinking or drug use?

G: Felt **G**uilty about the consequences of his or her drinking or drug use?

E: Taken a drink or drug in the morning as an "**E**ye opener" to decrease hangover or withdrawal?

A single positive response suggests that the clinician should exercise caution in prescribing opioids to the patient. This doesn't mean opioids are completely contraindicated, just that you should be especially careful in crafting your doctor/patient agreement (whether verbal or written), and you should pay particular attention to monitoring and follow-up. One of the most promising new tools for assessment of addiction is the Screener and Opioid Assessment for Patients in Pain (SOAPP) which offers a tool that focuses addiction screening directly toward the patient in pain. (This tool is available from the online pain education site www.painedu.org.)

2. Patient Education About Risks and Benefits of Therapy

For a host of reasons, any treatment for chronic pain should be the outcome of a conversation between you and your patient, and the treatment and treatment goals must be clearly understood and agreed upon. A treatment that is simply handed to a patient without his or her input, or which is hastily explained and possibly misunderstood by a patient is less likely to work or be adhered to.

How we position ourselves in the therapeutic decision-making process is also critically important. Since any beneficial treatment always carries some health risk, and the most aggressive treatments usually carry more risk, shared decision-making is critically important. It's the patient, after all, who will ultimately take on the work of adherence,[*] tolerating possible side effects, and the challenges of achieving functional improvement. A paternalistic approach where the clinician is all-knowing and is the sole decision maker may result in patient acceptance of the treatment without investment in full participation. If and when functional gains are not made, the head of this treatment regimen—the clinician—will then be responsible.

It is obviously best if the patient is put in charge and accepts ultimate responsible for him/herself. The clinician should serve as the expert advisor and consultant, but patients are best served by being put in the role of chief executive officer of their treatment regimens.

---

[*] The term "adherence" may be preferred to the more traditional "compliance" because of the possible connotations of coercion inherent in the word "compliance."

Patient adherence to any treatment regimen is directly related to their understanding of it, their belief that the treatment will do them good, and their motivation to tolerate or overcome any side-effects or adverse events related to the treatment. How you prepare a patient for a treatment, the degree to which you include him or her in decisions, and how you tie a treatment decision to the particulars of a patient's life are as important in the overall success of a treatment as the treatment itself.

Effective communication and patient education is also an integral part of "best practices" from both an ethical and a legal standpoint. A patient who does not fully understand the potential risks and benefits of a procedure or treatment cannot be said to be truly "informed." Inadequate education or communication on the part of a clinician, in other words, can have serious consequences.

I know how daunting the task of patient education can feel. Talking, listening, teaching, and assessing a patient's understanding of what we are saying unavoidably takes precious time. Some patients require more of your time than normal because they have so little background knowledge of how their own body works, or because they are stunned and perplexed by a chronic illness that confronts them with no risk-free option, including doing nothing. Sometimes the burden of education is not directly related to the pain. For instance, patients may not be native English speakers, or they may have learning disabilities of some kind. Other patients can demand our time for opposite reasons: they are so knowledgeable and articulate that they have highly technical or detailed questions and require similarly detailed answers. Or they may have read information from the Internet or other sources that is false or distorted and requires re-education. Or they are so anxious that they seem to have a never-ending stream of "what if" questions.

Patient education is both a big subject and a big business. Many programs and systems are sold to clinicians who are hungry for ways to make this process less time-consuming, more uniform, and more satisfying to patients. Such systems range in sophistication from sets of printed brochures to elaborate interactive programs using touch-screens and video presentations. A review of such programs is beyond the scope of this book, but clinicians who are intent on meeting the educational needs of their patients without adversely impacting their practice will have to embrace some system. Regardless of whether the system for educating patients is high or low tech, a well-made program that is flexible enough to respond to patients' unique questions and which can help document patient understanding of presented material can be a real help. But no program will ever—nor *should* ever—replace your face-to-face interaction with the patient.

Here are some strategies to make the communication of risks and benefits more time-efficient and still satisfying for patients:

Use Explanatory Hand-Outs about some of the basic ideas of pain management. These handouts can be given to patients either in the waiting room or by a nurse or other staff member in the examination room prior to your arrival—or on discharge pending a follow-up visit when the topic can be addressed after the patient had a chance to review the materials. Some of the topics in such handouts may include:

■ Basic categories of pain and its treatments.

■ Function-based perspective of pain treatment.

■ Basic risks and benefits of treatment, emphasizing that doing nothing *also* entails risk.

■ "Myths and Facts" about pain treatment in general (i.e., addressing patient fears that the doctor will think the pain is "all in their heads" or that they'll be seen as "weak").

■ Patient responsibilities and treatment expectations.

■ Potential drug side effects and signs that should warrant concern or action.

■ Administrative issues relating to your practice and how patients are expected to interface with your clinic.

Creating your own handouts may be the best option for any given practice and you can either start from scratch or mix and match from versions currently available online. (Education materials that you can download and print out may be obtained from the American Pain Foundation and the National Pain Foundation websites.) Regardless of the supporting materials you choose to use with your educational program, face-to-face time with your patient is critically important. You can keep you patients more engaged and receptive during this dialogue if you:

- **Stop frequently** to ask for questions and to check understanding.
- **Invite patients to interrupt** if they don't understand a word or phrase.
- **Prepare a list** of Internet sites or published resources such as consumer books on pain that you have reviewed and recommend for use by patients who seek more detailed explanations than you have time for. I often refer my patients to the American Pain Foundation (APF) or The National Pain Foundation (NPF) web sites, which have good patient support communities and offer extensive educational resources.

3. Clinician-Patient Treatment Agreements

Irrespective of whether or not you have a written agreement or simply have verbally come to a bilaterally agreed-upon course of treatment, you have a contract with your patient. Many clinicians feel that formalizing this process in writing offers clarity, consistency, durability, and efficiency. A written agreement should review all of the major points you have covered and agreed upon. Many pain management centers use an "opioid contract" as part of their standard practice when a patient is prescribed an opioid-containing medication. Some believe there is value in having consistency among *all* pain patients, and that a clear written understanding of the agreed-upon treatment regimen is more likely to enlist patient adherence, even in regimens that do not include opioids. Opioid prescribing may include more risk-management and monitoring obligations than non-opioid analgesic regimens, but any treatment regimen carries risks. Regardless of whether or not we are prescribing a drug that can be abused, there are tangible advantages to incorporating risk education information into a clear and transparent written document.

If you do use written agreements, be sure that the terms are completely acceptable to you and offer language that is consistent with your practice.

Crafting these agreements adds some up-front time to patient care but provides a number of advantages that I believe can benefit any patient and any treatment regimen. They can:

■ Help prevent misunderstandings or distortions of understanding over time.

■ Engage the patient in a collaborative decision-making process.

■ Serve as motivational reminders to the patient of the specific functional goals agreed upon with the clinician.

■ Serve as informed consent forms for a variety of treatment approaches. (Be sure to consult expert legal advice as to what constitutes informed consent in your state.)

■ Provide a foundation for later decision-making about changes in medications if functional goals are not achieved, or even if treatment is terminated if the patient fails to follow agreed-upon protocols (such as drug testing for patients taking opioids).

■ Enhance the therapeutic relationship between patient and doctor.

Of course, written agreements also provide some advantages to clinicians in terms of providing a written rationale for a treatment decision, evidence of patient education about risks, and proof of informed consent.

You can develop several types of agreements that are tailored for specific types of treatment and that include "open" areas to be filled in with the specific and unique aspects of the patient's treatment plan. For example, the list of functional goals can be either written in by hand or typed into a computer-based form and printed out for signing. At a minimum, any pain treatment agreement should include the following elements:

- Education about the risks and benefits of the specific agreed-upon treatment.
- Education about use of functional goals as guidelines for treatment decisions.
- Statement relating to individualized functional goals and agreed-upon processes for documenting progress.
- Need for patient to inform clinician of relevant information (i.e., side effects, medications, changes in condition).
- Statement of time course for the agreement.
- Terms about administrative expectations (such as, missed appointment, follow-up appointment, appearing without appointment, single pharmacy requirements, or expectations of how emergencies will be handled).
- Requirements for including or communicating with additional healthcare providers involved in care

(e.g., primary care clinician, physical therapist, or psychologist).

- Agreement issues (such as, who receives the agreement, and where the agreement is kept).
- Statement of patient privacy rights.
- Terms for administrative or other termination (e.g., abusing medication, missed appointments, violating agreement, inappropriate behavior, no improvement, pregnancy, tolerance, and toxicity).

If the treatment involves the use of opioid medications, the following elements may also be necessary:

- Patient responsibilities concerning improper use of controlled substances (includes overdosing, seeking medication elsewhere, selling medication, or stopping medication abruptly).
- Limitations for replacing lost medication or changing prescriptions.
- Limits on drug refills (phone allowances, only in person, call in advance, or during normal office hours).
- Agreement to submit to random drug screens.
- Education on side effects (including tolerance and withdrawal).
- Education on addiction risks and behaviors.
- Education on opioids and chronic pain.
- Pharmacy issues (one pharmacy, in-state pharmacy).
- Additional risks discussed (other drugs, masking conditions, misusing, or pregnancy).
- Need for single prescriber for all opioid prescriptions.

■ Dosing limitations and/or titration guidelines.
■ Terms concerning specific medications (such as, type prescribed, long-acting, or generic brands).

4. Monitoring Functional Progress, Adherence and Adverse Events

Your patient just left your office feeling hopeful that the pain will soon ease and that he or she will be able to begin the long process of recovery. You have listened carefully and have taken a thorough history. You've explained your approach and have agreed upon a set of functional goals. The treatments you've recommended are understood, including potential side effects and adverse events.

Now what? Is your job complete? Is recovery now the patient's responsibility?

Certainly your patients do bear a great deal of responsibility for their own healing. But you must monitor your patients' progress, be alert to undesirable or preventable side effects, and be sure they are advancing toward agreed-upon functional goals.

Monitoring progress toward functional goals is largely a matter of setting up attainable goals, with clear manifestations that the clinician can objectively gauge. The patient must bear the dual responsibility for attaining the goal as well as providing the required evidence of success. Without embracing both elements, functional outcomes become difficult to monitor and may fail. Regular visits with a patient are often needed and may require family members or friends to be included as collateral observers. Initially, it is important to set attainable functional goals and to try to stick to them. Flexibility is also required, however, so you can adjust goals either up or down in light of patient progress. As I noted in the previous chapter, objective outcomes can take many forms:

- Testimony by reliable partners or close friends who accompany the patient to appointments.
- Letters of acceptance into rehabilitation programs or support groups.
- Pay stubs from work.
- Bills from gyms, yoga programs, or other centers for conditioning.
- Ticket stubs from movies or musical performances.
- Photographs.

The evidence you request will vary with the patient, of course, and practical and clinical judgment will dictate what evidence will be necessary and how long, or to what degree, it will be needed. The important point is that patients are in charge of their therapy and part of their responsibility is to provide you with evidence of their progress. Meeting this part of the "deal" is a functional outcome in and of itself. If they are *unable* to document or achieve the progress outlined in your agreement, you will obviously need to reassess and make adjustments. (See the Monitoring section below for details.)

Monitoring adherence to medication regimens is an imperfect science, but it remains a valid and important part of therapeutic success. There are, at present, multiple ways to assess adherence, including simply asking about it, as well as by using diaries, written agreements, and laboratory screening. Effective adherence monitoring usually involves combining more than one of several simple low-cost techniques. Although a complete exploration of each of these adherence methods is beyond the scope of this book, I briefly review them here.

Traditional methods of measuring adherence to medical therapies include tablet counts, diaries, and patient interviews. Such methods have a number of advantages as well as drawbacks. Tablet counts are often unreliable because tablets may be discarded or possibly, in the case of opioids, hoarded, diverted, or sold. Containers can be lost or intentionally withheld. In addition, tablet counts offer no information about the pattern of medication use. Patient diaries are questionable representations of reality, particularly when reflecting use of opioids or any other potentially abusable or psychoactive drug. Patient interviews are subject to favorable bias on the part of the patient (i.e., forgetfulness, especially when the interval between drug use and interview exceeds two weeks).

Laboratory testing plays an important but partial role in the assessment of adherence.

Laboratory testing plays an important but partial role in the assessment of adherence. Such tests are often compromised by variability and limitations in obtaining specimens, custody of specimens, laboratory methodologies, and interpretation of laboratory data. Effective use of laboratory methodologies requires understanding many details of physiology, pharmacology, and toxicology—topics that are beyond the scope of this discussion. Most important, each laboratory uses different thresholds and standards that you will need to know before you'll be able to use their data with confidence.

For instance, in certain labs and for some drugs, only super-therapeutic values are reported. Thus, a patient might have a measurable level of a drug that is present but since it does not exceed the given threshold, it is reported as negative. In the case of a drug of abuse that might be diverted, misunderstanding the negative report to mean that no drug was present could have dire consequences. Knowing the laboratory protocol is necessary and, in the case described above where the lab reports only levels above a certain cut-off, the clinician should request reporting any measurable levels or a zero threshold. The presence and level of drugs can be detected in serum, urine, hair, and saliva. For routine drug surveillance, however, urine screening is most commonly used. Blood determination is not necessary in most clinical situations and many comprehensive toxicology laboratories are expanding their urine toxicology services and limiting serum analysis to special needs.

Urine is the standard and often exclusive specimen used in toxicology for routine drug surveillance of opioids or other monitored drugs. Advantages of urine testing include relative ease of sample acquisition, availability of a rapid, inexpensive, simple testing method, and longer duration of a positive result compared to that in serum. Unfortunately, urine screening is not perfect. Testing of opioid in urine is generally of two types: a screening method and a confirmatory test. Specimens found to be negative by the screening method usually require no further analysis. Positive samples may be further studied by a confirmatory test.

Confirmatory studies are necessary when the consequences of a false-positive result are significant, providing specific identification of individual opioid agents, such as morphine and codeine, rather than a class-specific opiate-positive finding. In such cases, it is advisable to use a laboratory that complies with the Substance Abuse & Mental Health Services Administration (SAMHSA) standards, and to use accepted chain of custody procedures for obtaining and handling the specimen.

If you suspect that a patient is non-adherent, you should never rush to judgment until you thoroughly investigate the underlying causes. Non-adherence may be related to any one of a long list of possibilities including adverse effects, forgetfulness, incompatibility with lifestyle, confusion about regimen, and so forth. It may rarely be related to aberrant behaviors such as diversion or drug abuse, and the astute clinician will maintain a position of vigilance without feeling compelled to reach immediate conclusions. In all cases, you must ensure that bias is not allowed to thwart appropriate medical care.

Be aware of the distinction between pseudo-addiction and true addiction. Patients who are receiving an inadequate dose of opioid medication often seek more pain medications to obtain pain relief. This is called pseudo-addiction because it is often mistaken for the true drug-seeking behavior of addiction. Other common signs of pseudo-addiction and inadequate analgesia may include:

- Requesting analgesics by name.
- Demanding, manipulative behavior.
- Clock watching (i.e., paying obsessive attention to when the next dose is scheduled).
- Taking opioid drugs for an extended period.
- Obtaining opiate drugs from more than one clinician.

Distinguishing between someone with addiction and pseudo-addiction can be challenging, and at times impossible on a single visit. This determination usually can only be made once the clinician prescribes an opioid that either improves or worsens function. Whereas pseudo-addiction resolves when the patient obtains adequate analgesia, true addictive behavior does not. Effectively treated patients experience improved function while arriving at dosages of medications that are stable and modulated. Patients who are addicted *don't* have improved function—typically their function decreases while aberrant behaviors suggest problems with modulating drug use.

The definition of drug addiction hinges on the compulsive use of a drug that causes harm or dysfunction, and the continued use despite that harm or dysfunction.

Patients with addiction have a disease that is stimulated by the drug that they are addicted to, resulting in dysfunction. Patients in pain are dysfunctional because of their pain, and the drugs that relieve their pain should improve their function. If you focus on function, these outcomes are diametrically opposite of each other.

Consultation with an addiction medicine specialist may be necessary at the point when you feel that true addiction may be a concern. Should you elect to pursue pain treatment with an abusable drug with a patient at documented risk for addiction, I suggest that you strongly consider working with an addiction specialist to ensure that you have the necessary resources to support an appropriate risk management program. As always, high vigilance and tempered judgment are required if the signs on the chart on page 82 are present, which may or may not indicate an abuse problem.

It's tempting to assume that patients with chronic pain who are not adherent to a treatment regimen are abusing medications. But other causes of non-adherence, such as those discussed above, must also be addressed. Once such causes have been eliminated, clear boundaries on prescribing may be in order. Use of the patient–clinician agreement can guide these decisions and make their implementation much less confrontational or controversial.

Modifying Treatments Over Time

Careful monitoring and thorough documentation will allow you to rationally and justifiably alter treatments as

(Behaviors **LESS** indicative of addiction)	(Behaviors **MORE** indicative of addiction)
1. Express anxiety or desperation over recurrent symptoms	1. Bought pain medications from a street dealer
2. Hoard medications	2. Stole money to obtain drugs
3. Taken someone else's pain medications	3. Tried to get opioids from more than one source
4. Aggressively complained to doctor for more drugs	4. Performed sex for drugs
5. Requested a specific drug medication	5. Seen two doctors at once or without them knowing
6. Used more opioids than recommended	6. Performed sex for money to buy drugs
7. Drink more alcohol when in pain	7. Stole drugs from others
8. Express worry over changing to a new drug even if it offers potentially fewer side effects	8. Prostituted others for money to obtain drugs
9. Taken (with permission) someone else's prescription opioids	9. Prostituted others for drugs
10. Raised dose of opioids on own	10. Prescription forgery
11. Expressed concern to clinician or family members that pain might lead to use of street drugs	11. Sold prescription drugs
12. Asked for second opinion about pain medications	
13. Smoke cigarettes to relieve pain	**Source:** Passik SD, Kirsh KL, Donaghy KB, Portenoy R. Pain and Aberrant Drug-Related Behaviors in Medically Ill Patients With and Without Histories of Substance Abuse. *Clin. J. Pain* 2006;22:173–181.
14. Ever used opioids to treat other symptoms	

needed. In all cases of a discrepancy between agreed-upon goals and the evidence of assessment, you need to carefully probe for the reasons behind the discrepancy. If functional goals are not being met, perhaps they were set too aggressively and need to be scaled back to allow the patient to have some "success" (as mentioned in the previous chapter). Perhaps the pain itself has not been lessened as much as needed. Perhaps there are motivational issues involved, such as a patient who has become so habituated to a passive existence that expending energy to become more active seems threatening or undesirable. In the case of a patient who is not meeting success, we must avoid the knee-jerk assumption that the patient is a failure. In such cases, I always ask myself if and how I may have set the care program up to fail and what changes might be made to facilitate success.

A common dilemma facing a diligent clinician is the situation of a patient who claims that increased activity is limited by increased pain. Since pain is neither measurable nor verifiable, how should a clinician respond? Rather than feeling forced to increase the dose of a medication, I suggest you take a step back and re-evaluate the functional goals. I have never met a person, even one who is dying, for whom increased function is not possible and beneficial. It all depends on how you define function. The dying patient may need to be able to wake up with reduced pain and be able to talk with a loved one. A patient with chronic pain may initially need an exceedingly gentle but persistent exercise plan.

The patient who says he or she can't exercise because of pain is almost always telling me that their exercise is starting at too intense a level. Finding the movement that does not cause pain may not be easy but it is possible. Doing that exercise for a while, and doing it repeatedly, can begin the conditioning process and allow for gradual increases in activity over time. After a while, the patient will become slightly more conditioned and able to gently expand the intensity. Remind patients that they are in a marathon, not a sprint. The "start low, go slow" protocol is, of course, easier to prescribe to another than accept for yourself—but it's a valid maxim and an important one to continually reinforce with your patients.

The number of ways a function-based treatment regimen can become derailed are practically infinite. But your fundamental response must always be the same:

■ Careful and compassionate listening.

■ Attention to the entire patient, not just to his or her pain.

■ Referral to related health professionals as needed to support a treatment plan (e.g., other medical specialists, mental health professionals, physical therapists, and social workers).

■ Adjustments to pain medications if indicated and reasonable in the larger context of everything you know about the patient's situation—but linking continuation of these medications to improvement in function or stabilization at an acceptable level.

- Modifications, if needed, to functional goals. Goals can be scaled back if progress is lacking, or can be made more aggressive if progress is rapid.
- Rewriting of the doctor/patient agreement as needed to reflect changes in treatment regimen, functional goals, or other aspects of the patient's condition.

Record-keeping systems that prepare for all of the updating variables may relieve much of the burden at the point of care. Standardized questionnaires can capture almost all critically important data. Among others, the Patient Assessment and Documentation Tool (PADT) is an excellent instrument for getting started (available from the National Pain Education Council website

Remind patients that they are in a marathon, not a sprint.

www.npecweb.org). The PADT offers a concise and time-efficient baseline for monitoring patients at follow-up visits, including pain, function, side effects, and aberrant behaviors. These data can be collected by office staff or patient; entries can be scanned into computers or entered directly by the patient through touch screens.

Chapter 4
Dealing With Difficult Patients

Pain upsets and destroys
the nature of the person who feels it.
— ARISTOTLE

I've had them. You've had them. Every clinician has had them: patients who can be deceitful, argumentative, manipulative, insulting, or just plain difficult. These patients are rare but when we do encounter them, they can take up a great deal of time and psychic energy. Patients dealing with chronic pain are often perceived as difficult and some can exhibit a range of diverse behaviors that can challenge the most poised and professional clinician. Patients in pain may have many reasons to be angry, argumentative, mistrustful, anxious, and depressed. (In my experience, depression and anxiety disorders are more prevalent among chronic-pain patients.)

These patients may strongly disagree with the clinician's assessment or treatment and can have idiosyncratic reactions to neural block procedures, such as a severe provocation of pain in the absence of any procedural complication. They can also display destructive behaviors, such as threats of suicide or self-mutilation, or demonstrate extreme noncompliance with treatment or opioid misuse. Even the most mild-mannered and polite person can become demanding and possibly even obnoxious under the lash of constant pain, sleep deprivation, hassles of traveling to the clinic, and frustration with physical limitations that make even the simplest activities, such as tying one's shoes, a struggle.

Aberrant behaviors do not exist in a vacuum, of course. Sometimes a clinician can introduce "difficulties" into the relationship as well. In the pressure-cooker of daily practice, it can be all too easy to lose our patience, our compassion, our warmth, and our sense of humor. Clinicians can be perceived as rude, arrogant, uncaring, disorganized, unintelligible, or rushed. Sometimes such perceptions are based on reality, sometimes not. But I have found that in any situation involving patient aberrant behavior, the source of the difficulty lies either in the patient, the clinician, or (most often) in a combination of patient/clinician personality attributes and the circumstances that have set up a dysfunctional dynamic.

An example from my own practice illustrates both of these points.

Mr. Smythe was a 58-year-old business executive recovering from open gall bladder surgery. Even before I saw Mr. Smythe, I heard him. As I was approaching his room I heard a man hurling insults at somebody, using language laced with four-letter words. I saw a nurse leave his room, scowling and obviously angry. When she saw me, she simply said, "I don't care what they say, I'm *not* trying to help that man again!"

I found Mr. Smythe glaring from his bed, which was surrounded by flowers and cards from well-wishers. He immediately launched into me.

"It's about time you showed up," he spat. "I'm in *!##/#* pain here and nobody's doing anything about it. And don't tell me I need more injections . . . I'm sick and tired of needles. If I don't get some relief soon you're going to hear from my lawyers."

Ordinarily I would have taken a deep breath and let his attitude and comments roll off my back. But this wasn't a good day for me. I had been working for 11 hours, I was hungry, and I was seriously behind on two grant applications due at the end of the week. I was simply in no mood to put up with abuse or threats.

"Look," I snapped. "Don't threaten me . . . I don't appreciate it."

He smirked. "Oh, you don't appreciate it," he said. "Well excuse me, Mr. Big Shot Doctor. You know what I don't appreciate? I don't appreciate loser doctors telling me they're going to stop my pain and then still hurting like hell."

We glared at each other, and I seriously considered walking out of the room. I was afraid that I'd say something I'd regret later. Then, from nowhere, I grinned.

"Then I guess we're even, aren't we?" I said. "I'll tell you what. I'll try to fix whatever is going wrong here if you'll just talk to me without swearing. Deal?"

He considered me for a moment. Then, gruffly, he said, "OK . . . deal."

I listened to his story. He had received multiple injections of morphine in his buttocks, which should have been more than enough to control his pain. (I have never understood why we continue to give patients intramuscular injections for pain—they are painful and there are other non-painful routes to use.) Nonetheless, something was interfering with the action of Mr. Smythe's analgesics. The lack of efficacy of his shots was clearly enough to transform this man into a behavioral cyclone. Mr. Smythe also mentioned some revealing personal background. He said he was the CEO of his business and was used to being in control. He hated feeling helpless and at the mercy of nurses and doctors half his age. In short, he was a classic "control freak" whose intense negative emotions surrounding receiving care were opposing the pharmacological effects of the morphine.

He was quite satisfied to be the CEO of his own pain regimen.

I decided to switch the delivery of his pain medication to a Patient Controlled Analgesic system. As soon as it was hooked up, he gave it a spin—several pushes over about 15 minutes. Over the next day, his distress was managed with far less morphine than his previous dosages and with less sedation and constipation. Moreover, he was quite satisfied to be the CEO of his own pain regimen.

Here was a patient with aberrant behavior and, at first, a clinician responding sub-optimally. Our initial stand-off could have escalated, leaving both of us angry and frustrated and him still in pain. Twenty-four hours later, however, Mr. Smythe was eating solid food, moving his bowels, chatting amiably with nurses, and making real progress toward discharge.

The Sources of Aberrant Behaviors

Individuals with chronic pain may be more likely to display aberrant behaviors because of the many psychosocial stressors that arise from pain and the impact of these stressors on mood, adjustment, coping, self-esteem, and personality. Chronic-pain patients often feel worthless, lonely, or abandoned, and they may become socially isolated and develop expectations of harm and disappointment. Some of these patients may have histories of childhood physical or sexual abuse or of underlying personality disorders that put them at risk for becoming increasingly anxious, dependent, obsessive, or paranoid. These psychological symptoms, in turn, may lead to distortions in sensory perception and amplification of pain.

Patients in pain can also be conflicted about whether or not they *want* the care they are offered. Such patients may simultaneously demand and reject care, simultaneously flattering and frustrating their clinicians. In mild cases, they make you uneasy; in extreme cases you may actually hate such patients or feel afraid of them.

Some of us find it difficult to acknowledge or discuss

such powerfully negative feelings. After all, we're not supposed to hate our patients—and most of us would simply rather not dislike anyone, most particularly one of our patients. But it's vitally important, both for ourselves *and* our patients that we become aware of our own emotional reactions to aberrant patient behavior, primarily so that we can control our responses. Denying our feelings may have been adaptive for many of us as we plodded through medical school and residencies, but this defense may become maladaptive in regular practice. If we are not aware of our own reactions or fail to understand them, we are apt to lack control, act impulsively, and make a tense situation worse.

When confronted with aberrant patient behavior, I am always helped by monitoring my own internal reactions which, I have learned, can serve as potential diagnostic data points. By paying attention to my emotional reactions, I can gain greater awareness, and bring much needed deliberation, planning, patience, and caution to a difficult situation, rather than acting from impulse or instinct. By adopting this perspective you may become the only member of a treatment team able to change the tide of acrimony surrounding a patient and re-establish effective treatment.

It's helpful to remember that if a patient is making you uncomfortable, he or she is probably even *more* uncomfortable—if not emotionally, then physically. The daily routines of hospital inpatients or of those housebound by pain can be arduous. One of my patients explained the "work" of chronic pain this way: "I can't button and unbutton my shirt. It's hard to comb my hair and hard to undress at night, and then I have to I wake up in the middle of the night to take the pain medication. Now I get constipated and have to take stuff for that. It's a hell of a lot of work."

We must appreciate the extent to which a patient's life is modified by a painful condition. All patients—but perhaps particularly those displaying aberrant behaviors—tend to feel relieved when their clinicians express interest in their lives. By framing their illness experience in terms of "work," you acknowledge the effort your patient is exerting in trying to heal, and you subtly reinforce the fact that they are, in the end, responsible for their own improvement.

Understanding why some patients behave in such a difficult manner, and perhaps how and why you react as well, may reduce your frustration and facilitate rational treatment. Often, these patients are extremely frightened or have low self-esteem. Such individuals often feel a persistent emptiness in their lives, and have labile moods and unstable personal relationships. Somewhat ironically, such patients often present with an affect of grandiosity, entitlement, or arrogance. Some may appear to have an almost carefree impassivity that is masking a distinct emotional fragility or tendency to be easily shamed or enraged. Challenging this entitled position usually serves only to confirm for patients that they are not receiving adequate attention, heightening their shame and humiliation, and intensifying their need for a demanding and entitled posture. While working with such patients, it is best to meet excessive demands with frequent and varied reminders that the patient deserves and will receive the best care possible.

Although each patient is unique, some astute clinicians have described discrete classes of patient aberrant behavior. Dr. James Groves,[*] for example, has identified some basic patient types that apply broadly in medicine, but which have particular relevance to those of us treating chronic pain:

■ **The Dependent Clinger.** These patients are often seductively grateful for your time and attention. They will flatter and sympathize even while they begin a steady escalation of their demands. An initially pleasant "honeymoon period" usually morphs into a time-consuming and emotionally corrosive relationship.

■ **The Entitled Demander.** These patients often arouse fear, anger, and guilt by their explicit or implicit message that "You guys are the doctors—why don't you know what's wrong and fix it?" Their entitlement often masks deep insecurity and self-doubt. The mantra of these patients is "I deserve your exclusive attention."

■ **The Manipulative Help Rejecter.** These patients are basically saying: "Help me, but you will fail." They may have no patho-physiological basis for their complaints and use their quest for an "accurate diagnosis" to certify and justify their lives. They may constantly seek that next clinician who will give them their next vague and untestable diagnosis. Participating in

---

[*] Groves, J.E. Management of the borderline patient on a medical or surgical ward. *Int. J. Psychiatry in Medicine*, 1975;6(3).

this dysfunctional pattern leads to perpetuation and frustration.

■ **Self-Destructive Deniers.** This is a relatively common type of patient, though only a minority of them will be dealing with chronic pain. Such patients intentionally or unintentionally persist in behaviors they know will eventually kill them: a patient with chronic obstructive pulmonary disease (COPD) who continues to smoke, a patient with liver disease who continues to drink alcohol, or a person with coronary artery disease who continues to eat fatty foods. Benevolent clinicians often feel conflicted by these patients—they can feel as though they're alone in trying to improve the patient's health and they can grow angry with patients who don't act in their own best interest and do not follow the clinician's advice.

Managing Aberrant Patient Behavior

The behaviors I discuss here are difficult because they challenge our psychic defenses, stretch our tolerance and patience, or demand much more of our time than we can give. It *is* possible to care for patients displaying such challenging behaviors, but only if you are first willing to recognize your own side of the equation.

Tuning in to your reactions is easier said than done. Aberrant behaviors such as manipulation, verbal abuse, or hostility almost dare us to make mistakes that we would never make in a normal non-threatening interaction. The most classic mistake is to just do something and get out—hoping that the patient will move on to somebody else who will take responsibility for his or her care. This is much like driving in a rain storm with dangerous slippery roads and instead of slowing down and driving slowly, you choose to speed up—thinking that the faster you go, the sooner you'll be out of the storm. But this is obviously a formula for disaster, either in a car or in the clinic with a difficult patient.

The only universal rule in these situations is to SLOW DOWN! Listen and watch more slowly and more purposefully than usual. Take your own pulse—ask why you are feeling this way and why you feel more strongly at this time than with other patients. Check your assumptions about the case and ask whether you are being pressured to do one thing or another without justification. Learn the different types of aberrant behaviors and watch for them—after a while, you will recognize them earlier in patient interactions. It will be like recognizing an old song—after only a few beats of the words or music, you can name the song, except in this case, you'll be quickly picking up on distinctive notes of dysfunction. As soon as you suspect something is not right, you need to slow down, take your time, and perhaps add a follow-up visit before jumping into therapeutic action. A common sense solution is usually available if you take the time to find it.

The only universal rule in these situations is to slow down!

Here are some practical rules of thumb for dealing with aberrant patient behaviors that I've developed over the years:

1. **Listen Closely** to the patient in order to determine his or her own understanding of the problem or disease, including any religious or cultural factors that might be influencing his or her beliefs about the problem or its potential treatment.

2. **Assume a Non-Confrontational Stance.** Dealing with a difficult patient can easily spiral into a battle of wills or wits that will solve nothing. Try to approach patients with the assumption that you are both on the same side. If they say or do things you disagree with or feel are groundless, pause and then reflect back to them what they just said rather than automatically rejecting, denying, dismissing, or contradicting. This takes practice and patience. If sometimes you "lose it" and find yourself stuck in a thicket of heated emotions, step back (literally, if necessary) and collect yourself. Nobody is perfect, but if you are willing to learn from your mistakes, you can progressively improve your practice.

3. **Take the Least Paternalistic Path** in your interactions. Remember that patients are in charge of their own health decisions. We are medical consultants. This means that the patient chooses to accept or reject what you offer, stay with you or see someone else. But you decide what to offer. I often say "I am your consultant, and I will give you my best advice but you must decide what to do." This shifts responsibility

and the direction of information flow from the perceived "omnipotent" clinician dictator who is telling the patient what to do to the "strong advisor" offering possible solutions for the client to adopt.

4. **Include the Patient** in planning the treatment regimen. The largest single determinant of the success of a treatment regimen may be a patient's ability and willingness to carry it out. Patients who participate in creating their treatment plan and who understand its underlying rationale are far more likely to adhere to it than those who are merely told what to do.

5. **Focus on the Big Picture.** Patients understandably focus narrowly on their pain, illness, or incapacitation and their words or actions arise from that tunnel vision. Clinicians can "pull back" to see not only the present situation, but the larger life context of the patient, antecedents that might be contributing to the problem, and the path from the present pain to a future function-based goal or outcome.

6. **Find and Agree on Common Goals** with the patient. If the goal is clinician-determined without input or assent from the patient, you'll be working at cross-purposes.

7. **Have Compassion.** One of the most concrete ways of demonstrating compassion is listening carefully and

with full attention, and interrupting only when the conversation loses focus. Each of us must find our own ways to let patients know that we are concerned—this is where the personality of the individual clinician will determine the approach.

8. **Set Limits for Acceptable Behavior.** No patient, regardless of the pain he or she may be in, has the right to insult, verbally abuse, threaten, or physically harm you. At the first instance of such behavior, you can say firmly and clearly that the behavior is unacceptable and if repeated, you will leave the room until the patient cools off. You could also turn care over to another clinician in such instances, since sometimes a different personality type may work better with certain patients. If patients threaten to harm themselves or others, they may need to be physically restrained and either the police or psychiatric assistance may be required. (Strictly adhere to any institutional policies in such cases.) Each of us should know our policies in this area and should think through plans of action if we find ourselves in an unsafe situation in our clinical practice.

9. **Call in a Pain Consultant**. Primary clinicians must both maintain an alliance with the difficult patient *and* set boundaries within which good healthcare can proceed and harm can be avoided. When the relationship becomes strained by constant demands or other

difficulties, it can be helpful to bring in a second party: a pain consultant who can offer an objective perspective and who is free of the long-term consequences of confronting mixed messages and inconsistent behaviors. Effective pain management consultants can offer strategies that preserve the self-esteem of both the patient and staff. The patient is best served when the consultant promotes the effectiveness of the primary team.

10. **Set Limits.** Setting limits on various aspects of the treatment plan may be a source of contention. In such cases, you should create an individualized plan based on rational treatment goals and back up the plan with an agreement—either formalized through a documented conversation, or in writing and signed by you and the patient. In all cases, you must not confuse limits with punishment or an opportunity for revenge. As difficult as it may be when confronted with hostility, denial, or manipulative behavior on the part of the patient, your treatment must be offered in a professional and kind manner, without malice or blaming.

Coping With Specific Aberrant Behaviors

The general guidelines I just described can be used in practically any situation involving aberrant behaviors. But some specific behaviors are common enough in the practice of pain medicine that they deserve some special mention.

Somatisizing Patients. Some patients believe they have a serious medical problem in the absence of demonstrable organic pathology. Usually these individuals believe their condition will get worse without treatment. They often have psychiatric comorbidity, and they portray their conditions as catastrophic and disabling. Clearly, since pain itself is untestable and the sources of pain can be legitimately obscure, we must be very cautious before concluding that a patient is somatisizing. Because somatization is ultimately a diagnosis of exclusion, I recommend that you take a patient's claims at face value during the initial phases of treatment, even if you harbor suspicions about their ultimate physical validity.

Take a patient's claims at face value even if you harbor suspicions about their ultimate physical validity.

If a program of functional evaluation and a treatment regimen using functional outcomes fails, and you continue to suspect somatization, you should consider referring the patient for a psychiatric consultation.

Hostile Patients. Occasionally patients will yell, be verbally abusive, or even physically threaten you or your staff. In these situations, try to maintain a relaxed posture and respect the patient's personal space. If I feel threatened, I share that with the patient. I'll say, "I'm feeling very threatened here, do I have a reason to worry?" I find that 99 percent of time when I let the patient *know* that I'm feeling threatened, the issue is defused. Usually, the patient isn't even aware that he or she is being threatening and he or she either apologizes or denies it but does, in fact, stop the threatening behavior.

Try to balance the need to handle hostile or threatening situations in private (an exam room or office, for instance) with the need to avoid too much isolation in situations in which your personal safety is in any question. If necessary, sit close to the door and possibly even keep the door open. Let others know that you are in with a hostile and threatening patient and have a plan if problems arise. If personal harm is a concern, in advance, ask security personnel or clinic staff to be present outside your exam room while you see the patient.

Irrespective of your concerns, you should strive to listen actively to the patient's complaints, maintain eye contact, and let the patient vent without interruption. After the encounter is over (whether or not an agreement or satisfactory closure has been possible), document the episode.

The suggestions I've just made are summed up in the "Five A's" below.

The Five A's For Dealing With Hostile Patients.[*]
Acknowledge the problem.
Allow the patient to vent uninterrupted in a private place.
Agree on what the problem is.
Affirm what can be done.
Assure follow-through.

---

[*] Wasan, A.D. et al. *Regional Anesthesia and Pain Medicine*, Vol. 30, No. 2, March-April 2005.

Sometimes a satisfactory resolution to a hostile situation cannot be reached, and assistance from security or the police is needed. Only in situations of imminent self-harm or harm to others should you or your staff attempt to restrain a patient.

Patients Who Lie. Unfortunately, lying is an unavoidable aspect of human nature. Many patients lie, but only sometimes does a lie (or lies) represent a real threat to the therapeutic relationship and the effectiveness of a treatment regimen. If you suspect a patient is lying to you and you feel the issue is important, you must raise the issue directly. In doing this, I find it helpful to remember (and to remind the patient) that my role is that of a professional consultant, with the patient being in charge of ultimate decision-making. I am not a judge or jury. Though I might feel betrayed or angry at being deceived, my role is not to punish, but to present facts and find solutions. To that end, I might say to a patient, "You know, I might be wrong about this, but the information I have suggests that you aren't being honest with me, and I can't help you effectively if I can't trust you or trust what is happening in your therapy."

It can be difficult, but try to see a lie as data—it is telling you something about the patient. It's a "yellow light" signaling caution, and in and of itself does not require rejection or termination. Your task is to try to find the truth without stigmatizing or harming the patient, and without making yourself feel better at expense of the patient. (Some situations, of course, are intolerable and certain lies are not acceptable. See the section below on terminating care.)

Patients You Suspect of Addiction. Earlier in this book I talked about the need to differentiate between true addiction and pseudo-addiction, which is drug-seeking behavior that arises from a desire for increased symptom control and which, in fact, does result in better functioning. Patients who are truly addicted can be deceptive and manipulative. For example, they may express concern or even horror over taking an opioid-containing medicine, but will then maneuver to make opioids appear to be the lesser of evils. A wide range of aberrant behaviors can be mistaken for signs of addiction, such as a patient who unilaterally raises his or her dose of an opioid, or who uses a friend's medication. Most often, however, these behaviors are "yellow lights" signaling caution, rather than "red lights" signaling addiction and a need for immediate prescription termination.

Non-adherent behavior is seen amongst patients in all aspects of medical care, not just in pain management. When it occurs with opioids or other abusable prescription medications, we must be careful to remember that the behaviors may stem from many different etiologies, from addiction and diversion to untreated pain and psychological distress, to name a few. In my experience, opioid-treated, chronic pain patients are frequently non-adherent, but only a small minority of these patients are truly addicted. This means that "one strike and you're out" policies are misguided and excessively punitive. The patient who flunks a urine test, runs out of a prescription early, or complains aggressively should not simply be kicked out and denied medication. I recommend using all of the therapeutic skills I have reviewed earlier to understand the problem, listen to the patient, and find a function-based solution. Remember that you are the consultant and not the parent, priest, rabbi, judge, or jury. Even when one line of therapy may no longer be safe or appropriate for a given patient, there may be other treatments that we can offer.

Terminating a Relationship

Aberrant patient behaviors will rarely require that the patient be dismissed or "fired" from a practice. You can, and should, have a "zero tolerance" policy for any illegal behavior (selling prescription medications, threatening violence, or forging clinician signatures, for example). Other situations can make "administrative termination" necessary as well, such as an opioid-addicted patient who refuses treatment for his or her addiction and continues to ask for prescriptions.

In such cases, I recommend that you first inform the patient of the reasons you can no longer treat him or her. You should, preferably, do this during a face-to-face visit and follow up with a formal letter. In the absence of a face-to-face meeting, a certified letter may be necessary. You can specify the terms of separation such as stating that, 30 days after receiving the letter, the patient will no longer be admitted to your practice. Determining exactly how to achieve the best result for the patient and yourself, however, will require individualization. All clinicians are bound by an ethical duty not to abandon a patient. Exactly how you fulfill this responsibility may also require professional consultation. In most situations, you may give the patient names of other providers or contact information for the local medical society, from which he or she can obtain a list of other providers. Last, at discharge, you may need to consider how the patient will tolerate discontinuation without harm, and in cases involving opioids, benzodiazepines, anticonvulsants, or antidepressants, among others, safe discontinuation may require a tapering schedule.

The Rewards of Perseverance

Managing aberrant patient behavior is certainly challenging, but it can also be rewarding. As we've seen, a very few patients may push so far beyond the bounds of acceptable conduct that you need to sever your relationship with them. Most difficult behaviors, however, will be found upon compassionate reflection to be rooted in patient fear, frustration, anxiety, past trauma, or simply the corrosive effects of fatigue and stress.

In many ways, the patients displaying the most severe behaviors are the ones most in need of our help. Such patients can challenge our self-image as a nurturing care giver. When I feel hostility or even hatred toward a difficult patient, I often recall the truism that the opposite of love is not hate, but indifference. Resenting a difficult patient is proof that you care about his or her welfare and are frustrated that you can't resolve the conflicts that are getting in the way of therapy. Don't beat yourself up for being "uncaring," since it is only from your caring nature that your strong feelings emerge.

Disliking or hating a patient is never comfortable, but it's important not to deny those feelings to yourself. Self-awareness will offer you the tools to gain control and retain the elements of care that make you an effective clinician.

If you approach aberrant behavior with frustration, confrontation, or negative emotions, you will most likely hasten the deterioration of an already strained relationship. On the other hand, if you take your pulse and your time, you will find common sense solutions that were previously obscured by emotion. You may also create a "space" for the better aspects of any patient's personality to manifest themselves, which will benefit everyone. In the best case scenario—and yes, this happens sometimes with even the most difficult patients—you may be rewarded with the gratitude of patients who, despite some lingering behavior issues, nonetheless become willing and productive partners in their own healthcare.

If you take your pulse and your time, you will find common sense solutions that were previously obscured by emotion.

LISTENING TO PAIN

Chapter 5
Clinician Survival

Straining breaks the bow,
and relaxation relieves the mind.

— SYRUS (PUBLILIUS SYRUS), *Maxims*

I usually get a smile when I present the following two maxims of clinical practice related to patients in chronic pain:

1. The clinician must have less pain than the patient.
2. The clinician must survive.

Unfortunately, I'm not actually joking. In order to give to others, we must be careful to take care of ourselves. Clinicians are surrounded by stressors, whether from patients, regulators, lack of time, or demands outside of our professional lives. We cannot help a patient in pain if such stressors are generating even greater "pain" for us. We cannot be effective clinicians if we become so burned out that we're simply going through the motions of patient care. In short, we must survive emotionally if we're to be of any benefit to our patients.

In the prior chapter I highlighted a variety of difficult patients and difficult situations you're likely to have to cope with in the course of treating patients in pain, and the emotional toll they can take on us. What I didn't say is that treating pain patients itself can be exhausting. In order to treat pain, you have to engage with the lives of people in pain and the suffering they're experiencing. Not only do we have to face the pain our patients are experiencing, but we must also confront the truth that sometimes we can't relieve their suffering, that there are usually no quick fixes for pain, and often no cure for the underlying condition that's causing the pain. Working so hard to relieve patients' suffering—often with only partial success—can easily fill us with a feeling of futility that can lead to burnout.

Where you turn to find the strength and resilience to remain effective as a clinician is a deeply personal question, and for many of us, a fundamentally spiritual one. I'm a clinician, not a chaplain, so let me offer some practical advice, as well my personal perspective as a pain medicine specialist.

First, cut yourself some slack. If you're like most doctors, you were trained to view success in terms of curing or defeating a disease. Chronic pain doesn't lend itself well to win/lose scenarios, and as we've discussed previously, vanquishing pain altogether isn't the goal. The goal is relieving your patient's suffering, and often relieving suffering has less to do with analgesia than with restoring meaningful function and quality of life. In the same way that we need to shift our patient's focus from pain relief to functional goals and outcomes, as doctors we have to refocus and redefine our own definition of "success." We may not be able to stop the pain, but in 9 cases out of 10, we can do something meaningful to improve a patient's quality of life—and we should allow ourselves to take satisfaction from that accomplishment.

But what about the patients who don't improve under our care? What about the chronically ill or chronically in-pain patient who spirals down into total incapacity? What about a cancer patient who is dying, despite our best efforts to manage his or her pain? How do we defend ourselves against despair in the face of suffering we can't prevent?

As any behavioral therapist would tell you, it helps to share your frustration and feelings of futility with your peers and colleagues. They'll understand what you're going through and their understanding will help ease your pain. It will also make them feel better—they'll realize that they're not alone in their feelings of helplessness, and they'll know that they too have someone to turn to. Again, we're not trained in medical school or residency to admit "defeat" or despair to our colleagues. We're trained to "consult" with each other, but not to confide. But after years of running training programs and pain services, I've learned the irreplaceable value of fostering a caring community of clinicians who can support each other and share the emotional burden of treating suffering in an increasingly difficult medical environment. The more we can share—not just about our patients' morbidity and mortality, but about our own frailty—the more resilient we become as individuals and as a group. Without resilience we can't expect to have the emotional and physical stamina we need to be caring and effective pain managers.

Some doctors turn to their spouses to help absorb the stress of their work—but I've also seen that strategy backfire by putting a lot of stress on the marriage, which creates a different kind of burnout. My advice to residents and fellows is: even if you have a very understanding spouse or partner at home, make sure you also have a supportive community of peers—even if it's only a colleague or two—with whom you can share the frustrations, fears, and joy of your work.

But in the end, it's not going to be your colleagues or your spouse who's going to be your source of renewal, who's going to give you the energy and enthusiasm you need to return to work every morning in this most demanding of professions. For that, you'll have to turn to . . . your patients.

That's right. As paradoxical as it sounds, your most reliable source of strength can be the same patients in pain who can drive you to distraction and to the brink of exhaustion—*if you have the courage to connect with them.* If you avoid their pain, or look past their suffering, they'll only further drain your batteries. But if you face them openly and with compassion, the part of you that's depleted and wounded will be refilled and restored. Because that connection and compassion will be as therapeutic for your patients as any drug trial and, in some cases, will be the difference between therapeutic success and failure. And when your patients improve, so will your spirits.

Last year, I had my first sabbatical from my job at the University of California, Davis School of Medicine where I teach, do research, and run a large clinical pain service. I knew I'd miss the teaching, but I was looking forward to being free from the demands of my clinical practice so I could spend more time on research and writing. But what I discovered is that, in a way I had not anticipated, I missed my patients. Even though I had fewer clinical and academic responsibilities during my sabbatical year—to residents, to colleagues and especially to patients—and even though I was as busy as ever, engaged in legislative and advocacy activities of importance to the field of pain medicine, I felt a void. I realized that though I have an over-scheduled and over-committed work life, it's the daily interaction with my patients that grounds me.

This may seem surprising since many of my patients are the most difficult in our clinic. It is actually surprising to me, too—but in all the hub-bub and consternation that difficult patients can bring to a clinical visit, being the person with whom they can forge a productive therapeutic relationship is deeply gratifying. What I've learned over time is to see the big picture and to cut the best deal possible with the patients and the bureaucracy that will best meet their needs. But the biggest reward is being able to offer them connection when all they have known is a fragmented medical world that serially rejects them because they are a difficult case or have a difficult personality. My job is to stay in the game and stay functional in the process.

Sure, there are patients whose mere name on a chart makes me cringe, patients who make me want to turn and flee on sight. But every time I manage to face them and their suffering head-on with compassion, and I am able to reach them, I feel renewed. I remember why I went to medical school in the first place, why I wanted to be a pain medicine specialist, and why I am able to reclaim the passion to heal every time I walk into my clinic.

I'm convinced that the rewards of treating pain are available to every clinician. You don't have to be the best communicator or have the warmest bedside manner. All you need is the desire to relieve suffering and the understanding that an important part of making the pain stop is simply showing up and showing your patients that you care. Some of us do it with our voices, some with the healing touch of our hands, some with our sense of humor. Sometimes it's simply having the guts to look patients in the eye and acknowledge their pain. They feel less alone. They feel cared for and healed. And in a mysterious and powerful way, so do we.

Appendix
Resources for Pain Management

As with any job, effectively treating patients in chronic pain is easier when you use the right tools. I'm talking here about assessment instruments, scales for quantifying pain, intake questionnaires, patient education handouts, and well-crafted doctor/patient agreements. Many versions of these kinds of tools are available for downloading from the Internet. Below I've listed the sites I can recommend to you—and I've marked my most highly recommended sites with a ✪. I've also listed some books about pain and pain management that you or your patients might find helpful.

1. **Medical Specialty Society Sites**
2. **Nonprofit Pain Organizations (and other sites of interest to medical professionals)**
3. **Pain and Function Assessment Tools**
4. **Medical Journals Focusing on Pain**
5. **Sites with Educational Information for Consumers**
6. **Professional and Patient Sites by Disorder**
7. **Pain-Related Books**

1. Medical Specialty Society Sites

American Academy of Orofacial Pain
www.aaop.org
19 Mantua Road
Mount Royal, NJ 08061
856/423-3629
Fax: 856-423-3420

✪ The American Academy of Pain Medicine
www.painmed.org
4700 W. Lake Ave.
Glenview, IL 60025
847/375-4731
Fax 847/375-4777

American Medical Association
www.ama-assn.org
515 N. State Street
Chicago, IL 60610
(800) 621-8335

✪ American Pain Society (APS)
www.ampainsoc.org
4700 W. Lake Ave.
Glenview, IL 60025
847-375-4715
Fax: 877-734-8758

A multidisciplinary organization of basic and clinical scientists, practicing clinicians, policy analysts, and others. The mission of the APS is to advance pain-related research, education, treatment, and professional practice.

American Psychological Association

www.apa.org
750 First Street, NE
Washington, DC 20002
Telephone: 800-374-2721
Offers referrals, assistance, and resources for coping with the psychological aspects of trauma and terrorism.

American Society of Addiction Medicine

www.asam.org
Email@asam.org
4601 North Park Ave, Arcade Suite 101
Chevy Chase, M.D. 20815
301/656-3920
Fax 301/656-3815

American Society for Pain Management Nursing

www.aspmn.org
7794 Grow Drive
Pensacola, FL 32514
888/34-ASPMN (342-7766)
Fax 850/484-8762

American Society of Regional Anesthesia and Pain Medicine
www.asra.com
P.O. Box 11086
Richmond, VA 23230-1086
804/282-0010
Fax 804/282/0090

2. Nonprofit Pain Organizations (and other sites of interest to medical professionals)

American Council for Headache Education
www.achenet.org
19 Mantua Road
Mt. Royal, NJ 08061
Tel: 856-423-0258 800-255-ACHE (255-2243)
Fax: 856-423-0082

✪ **AMA Pain Management: The Online Series**
www.ama-cmeonline.com
Web-based Continuing Medical Education program on pain management from the American Medical Association

✪ **American Pain Foundation**
www.painfoundation.org
info@painfoundation.org
201 North Charles Street
Suite 710
Baltimore, MD 21201-4111

Tel: 888-615-PAIN (7246)
Fax: 410-385-1832
An excellent source for patient information and advocacy.

Arthritis Foundation
www.arthritis.org
help@arthritis.org
1330 West Peachtree Street
Suite 100
Atlanta, GA 30309
Tel: 800-568-4045 404-872-7100 404-965-7888
Fax: 404-872-0457

City of Hope Pain/Palliative Care Resource Center
www.cityofhope.org/prc/
City of Hope Pain/Palliative Care Resource Center
Duarte CA

City of Hope Pain Resource Center: Nursing Research and Education (COHPPRC)
www.cityofhope.org/prc/
A clearinghouse of resources to enable individuals and institutions to improve the quality of pain management. This site has wealth of information for patients, including a question-and-answer series by Dr. Fishman, as well as extensive links to further information for consumers.

The Cochrane Collaboration
www.cochrane.org
A wide-ranging collection of evidence-based reviews.

Fibromyalgia Network
www.fmnetnews.com
Educational materials on fibromyalgia syndrome
(FMS) and chronic fatigue syndrome (CFS).

International Association for the Study of Pain
www.iasp-pain.org
The leading international society of pain professionals; its
website offers many valuable resources for professionals.

The Mayday Pain Project
www.painandhealth.org
Internet links and resources.

National Consensus Project for Quality Palliative Care
www.nationalconsensusproject.org
A collaborative project of the American Academy of
Hospice and Palliative Medicine, Hospice and
Palliative Nurses Association, and the National
Hospice and Palliative Care Organization to promote
the implementation of Clinical Practice Guidelines for
new and existing palliative care services.

National Institute of Dental and Craniofacial Research (NIDCR)
www.nidcr.nih.gov
nidcrinfo@mail.nih.gov
National Institutes of Health, DHHS
31 Center Drive, Room 5B-55
Bethesda, MD 20892

National Headache Foundation
www.headaches.org
info@headaches.org
820 N. Orleans
Suite 217
Chicago, IL 60610-3132
Tel: 312-274-2650 888-NHF-5552 (643-5552)
Fax: 312-640-9049

Penn Center for Bioethics
www.bioethics.upenn.edu/
A general introduction to bioethics, including a listing
of related external links and organizations.

TALARIA Guidelines for Cancer Pain
www.talaria.org

UCLA History of Pain Project: The John C. Liebskind History of Pain Collection

www.library.ucla.edu/libraries/biomed/his/pain.html
The most exstensive resource on the historical aspects of pain.

University of Wisconsin Pain and Policy Studies Group

www.medsch.wisc.edu/painpolicy/
A good resource for pain-related public policy and legislative issues.

3. Pain and Function Assessment Tools

The assessment tools below are widely available online for downloading in various formats, including at several of the commercially sponsored sites described in Section 5.

Initial Pain Assessment Tool

www3.mdanderson.org/depts/prg/bpi.htm
A charting form that can be used on the patient's initial admission to document location, intensity, quality of pain, and relief.

Brief Pain Inventory (BPI)

www.cityofhope.org/prc/pdf/BPI%20Short%20Version.pdf
A brief, simple, and easy to use tool for the assessment
of pain in both clinical and research settings. The BPI
uses simple numeric rating scales from 0 to 10 that are
easy to understand and easy to translate into other lan-
guages. It is a well-validated instrument to measure pain
intensity, functionality, and the impact of pain on one's
life in the past 24 hours and within the past week.

McGill Pain Questionnaire

www.cityofhope.org/prc/pdf/McGill%20Pain%
20Questionnaire.pdf
A 20-item scale that allows patients to articulate
ranges of pain sensation, both internal and external.

Visual Analog Scale

www.ndhcri.org/pain/Tools/Visual_Analog_Pain_Scale.pdf
A linear scale from Worst Imaginable Pain to No Pain.
Patients place a mark along the line to indicate their
current pain level.

Wong-Baker FACES Pain Rating Scale
www3.us.elsevierhealth.com/WOW/

A scale that employs pictures of faces, ranging from happy
to sad to assess pain in children; while designed to assess
pain in children; it is also used to assess pain in adults.

4. Medical Journals Focusing on Pain

Headache: The Journal of Head and Face Pain
American Headache Society
www.blackwellpublishing.com/journal.asp?ref=0017-8748

Journal of Pain
American Pain Society
http://journals.elsevierhealth.com/periodicals/yjpai

Journal of Pain and Symptom Management Pain
International Association for the Study of Pain
www.elsevier.com/homepage/sah/pain/menu.html

Pain Medicine
American Academy of Pain Medicine
www.blackwellpublishing.com/journal.asp?ref=1526-2375&site=1

Pain Research and Management
Canadian Pain Society
www.pulsus.com/pain/home.htm

Revista De La Sociedad Española Del Dolor
http://wwwscielo.isciii.es/scielo.php/script_sci_serial/pid_1134-8046/lng_en/nrm_iso

5. Sites with Educational Information for Consumers

✪ **American Pain Foundation**
www.painfoundation.org
info@painfoundation.org
201 North Charles Street
Suite 710
Baltimore, MD 21201-4111
Tel: 888-615-PAIN (7246)
Fax: 410-385-1832
An excellent source for patient information and advocacy.

6. Professional and Patient Sites by Disorder

ARTHRITIS

Arthritis Foundation
www.arthritis.org

Medical College of Wisconsin/Arthritis
healthlink.mcw.edu/arthritis/

Mayo Clinic Arthritis Center
www.mayoclinic.com/health/arthritis/AR99999

BACK AND SPINE PAIN

Spine Health
www.spine-health.com

Spine Universe
www.spineuniverse.com

CANCER PAIN

The American Alliance of Cancer Pain Initiatives (AACPI)
www.aacpi.wisc.edu
1300 University Avenue, Room 4720
Madison, WI 53706
(608)265-8656
Fax: (608)265-4014

American Cancer Society
www.cancer.org

Cancer Pain Control:
www.WHOcancerpain.wisc.edu

The Cancer Pain Education Resource (CAPER)
www.caper.tufts.edu

City of Hope Pain/Palliative Care Resource Center
www.cityofhope.org/prc

FIBROMYALGIA PAIN

The American Fibromyalgia Syndrome Association
www.afsafund.org

Fibromyalgia Network
www.fmnetnews.com

National Fibromyalgia Association
http://fmaware.org

HEADACHE PAIN

National Headache Foundation
www.headaches.org

American Council for Headache Education
www.achenet.org

TMJ Tutorial
www.rad.washington.edu/anatomy/modules/TMJ/TMJ.html

COMPLEX REGIONAL PAIN (CRPS) PAIN INTERNET RESOURCES

Reflex Sympathetic Dystrophy Syndrome Association of America
www.rsds.org

American RSDHope Group
www.rsdhope.org

NINDS Complex Regional Pain Syndrome Information Page from the National Institute of Neurological Disorders and Stroke
www.ninds.nih.gov/disorders/reflex_sympathetic_
dystrophy/reflex_sympathetic_dystrophy.htm

PEDIATRIC PAIN

American Academy of Pediatrics
www.aap.org

KidsHealth
www.kidsheath.org

Pediatric Pain—Science Helping Children
www.dal.ca/~pedpain/pedpain.html

7. Pain-Related Books
(available at amazon.com and other online bookstores)

The Body in Pain: *The Making and Unmaking of the World*
Elaine Scarry (Oxford University Press 1985).

Cancer Pain Relief
International Association for the Study of Pain; World
Health Organization, (World Health Organization 1986).

***Cancer Pain Relief and Palliative Care: Report of a
WHO Expert Committee, WHO Technical Report
Series 804***
World Health Organization (World Health
Organization 1990).

Core Curriculum for Professional Education in Pain
International Association for the Study of Pain, Task Force
on Professional Education, (IASP Publications 1991).

The Culture of Pain
David B. Morris (University of California Press 1993).

Dying Well: Peace and Possibilities at the End of Life
Ira Byock (Riverhead 1998).

***Full Catastrophe Living: Using the Wisdom of Your
Body and Mind to Face Stress, Pain, and Illness***
Jon Kabat-Zinn (Delta 1990).

Handbook of Cancer Pain Management 3rd Edition
Weissman et al. (Wisconsin Pain Initiative 1992).

How We Die: Reflections on Life's Final Chapter
Sherwin B. Nuland (Vintage 1995).

*The Illness Narratives: Suffering, Healing, and the
Human Condition*
A. Kleinman (Basic Books 1988).

Managing Pain Before It Manages You
Margaret A. Caudill (Guilford Press 2001).

*Mastering Pain: A Twelve-Step Program for Coping
With Chronic Pain*
Richard A. Sternbach (Putnam 1987).

*Natural Pain Relief: A Practical Handbook
for Self-Help*
Jan Sadler, Patrick Wall (C.W. Daniel Company 2004).

Nature of Suffering and the Goals of Medicine
Eric J. Cassell (Oxford University Press, USA 2004).

On Death and Dying
Elisabeth Kubler-Ross (Scribner 1997).

Pain and Suffering
William K. Livingston, Howard L. Fields (IASP Press 1998).

Phantoms in the Brain: Probing the Mysteries of the Human Mind
V. S. Ramachandran, Sandra Blakeslee (Harper Perennial 1999).

Principles & Practice of Pain Management
Carol A Warfield, Zahid H. Bajwa (McGraw-Hill Professional Publishing; 2nd edition 2003).

Suffering
Betty Ferrell, Editor (Jones & Bartlett Publishers 1996).

The War on Pain
Scott Fishman (Harper Paperbacks 2001).

When Bad Things Happen to Good People
Harold S. Kushner (Anchor 2004).

Wherever You Go, There You Are: Mindfulness Meditation in Everyday Life
Jon Kabat-Zinn (Hyperion 2004).

Acknowledgments

This book was written to help primary care clinicians and other specialists meet the pain management needs of their patients at a time when under-treatment of pain has become a public health crisis.

Stephen Braun, an experienced and talented medical editor and writer, made significant contributions to the manuscript. Beginning with conceptual conversations about each chapter and ending with meticulous line editing, Stephen performed much of the heavy spadework and delicate pruning involved in creating this book. He has my thanks and appreciation. This book was originally produced at Waterford Life Sciences, and I thank Josh Horwitz, publisher at Waterford, for sharing my enthusiasm for this project and skillfully bringing the project to fruition. I also thank Gretchen Maxwell and Kate Lessing for their design and copyediting talents as well as Marlene Mascioli and Dr. Janelle Guirguis-Blake for their invaluable help in reviewing and finalizing the manuscript.

I could have not have produced this book without the support of my colleagues at the Division of Pain Medicine of the University of California, Davis, who, on a daily basis, provided me with a rare and invaluable professional community. They include my remarkable clinician partners Drs. Paul Kreis, Gagan Mahajan, Ingela Symreng, David Copenhaver, Samir Sheth, Naileshni Singh, Robert McCarron, Peter Moore, and many others. I am indebted to Jan Aaron, who guided our division for many years but succumbed to cancer at the time that this book was completed. Jan made my work a joy and is sorely missed.

I am truly blessed with a wonderful family who graciously endure the demands of my work. They complete my life beyond words.

Finally, I am beholden to all of my patients who enhance my life by sharing theirs with me and who never cease to convince me of the power of the human spirit.

About the Author

Scott M. Fishman, M.D., is a nationally recognized author and advocate for patients in pain. He is chief of the Division of Pain Medicine and Professor of Anesthesiology and Pain Medicine at the University of California, Davis. He was formally medical director of Massachusetts General Hospital Pain Center at Harvard Medical School. Dr. Fishman was trained and board certified in Internal Medicine, Psychiatry, Pain Medicine, and Hospice and Palliative Care.

Dr. Fishman lectures on all aspects of pain control as well as on the risks of prescription drug abuse throughout the United States. He authored *Responsible Opioid Prescribing* for the Federation of State Medical Boards, which has been delivered to over 200,000 US prescribers through 20 state medical boards. He has also authored *The War on Pain* (Harper Collins), co-authored *Spinal Cord Stimulation: Implantation Techniques* (Oxford University Press), and co-edited *Bonica's Management of Pain* 4th ed. (Lippincott), *The Massachusetts General Hospital Handbook of Pain Management* 2nd ed. (Lippincott), and *Essentials of Pain Medicine and Regional Anesthesia* (Elsevier). Dr. Fishman has authored many peer-reviewed articles in medical journals, book chapters, and other scholarly reviews. He is senior editor of the journal *Pain Medicine* and serves on the editorial board of other medical journals.

Dr. Fishman is past president and past chairman of the board for the American Pain Foundation. He is also past president of the American Academy of Pain Medicine and previously served on the board of directors for the American Pain Society. He advocates for safe and effective pain control with consumers and lawmakers, having testified in both state and national legislatures and consulted with numerous government agencies and organizations.

CPSIA information can be obtained at www.ICGtesting.com
Printed in the USA
BVOW072011120112

280306BV00001B/3/P